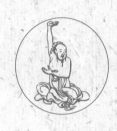

U0334984

中医养生功法（汉英对照）
Chinese Medical Qigong Exercises for Nurturing Life
(*Chinese-English Edition*)

八段锦
Ba Duan Jin

魏玉龙　编著
Written by Wei Yulong
沈　艺　张晓枚　译
Translated by Shen Yi and Zhang Xiaomei

全国百佳图书出版单位
中国中医药出版社
·北京·

China Press of Traditional Chinese Medicine
· Beijing ·

图书在版编目（CIP）数据

八段锦：汉英对照 / 魏玉龙编著；沈艺，张晓枚译 .—北京：
中国中医药出版社，2021.6
ISBN 978 – 7 – 5132 – 6768 – 7

Ⅰ . ①八… Ⅱ . ①魏… ②沈… ③张… Ⅲ . ①八段锦—
基本知识—汉、英 Ⅳ . ① G852.9–64

中国版本图书馆 CIP 数据核字（2021）第 038365 号

中国中医药出版社出版

北京经济技术开发区科创十三街 31 号院二区 8 号楼
邮政编码　100176
传真　010–64405721
河北新华第二印刷有限责任公司印刷
各地新华书店经销

开本　880×1230　1/32　印张 5　字数 132 千字
2021 年 6 月第 1 版　2021 年 6 月第 1 次印刷
书号　ISBN 978 – 7 – 5132 – 6768 – 7

定价　39.00 元
网址　www.cptcm.com

社 长 热 线　010–64405720
购 书 热 线　010–89535836
维 权 打 假　010–64405753

微信服务号　zgzyycbs
微商城网址　https://kdt.im/LIdUGr
官 方 微 博　http://e.weibo.com/cptcm
天猫旗舰店网址　https://zgzyycbs.tmall.com

如有印装质量问题请与本社出版部联系（010–64405510）
版权专有　侵权必究

导　言

八段锦①是当下国际上普及最为广泛的中国古代传统养生康复的代表功法之一，其动作舒展大方，尤其以人体的脊柱为中心，是左右对称、前后协调、上下协同的操作技巧，通过对机体持续、整体的训练，达到通行全身气血、强身健体的养生康复作用和目的。

八段锦的历史久远、影响深远，其操作方法和养生理念最早可追溯到上古时期的尧舜时期，源于部落先民舒展肢体训练对"湿气②"致病的防治。其多个动作可以在汉代的导引图中找到操作原型，而其动作的初步形成被记录在南朝梁代陶弘景著的《养性延命录》中。"八段锦"的这一名称最早见于南宋洪迈的《夷坚志》，而整套功法的最早文字记录则见于南宋曾慥的《道枢·众妙篇》。现在流行的动作歌诀最早见于宋元时期的《灵剑子导引子午诀》，至明末清初，基本定型成为八段锦功法各节的名称沿用至今。歌诀是这样表述的，"两手托天理三焦，左右开弓似射雕，调理脾胃须单举，五劳七伤往后瞧，摇头摆尾去心火，两手攀足固肾腰，攒拳怒目增气力，背后七颠百病消"。

八段锦属于中国古代传统锻炼技术的范畴，而中国古代传统锻炼技术包含调身（姿势动作的训练）、调息（呼吸运动的训练）、调心（心理状态的训练）三个要素。历代文献对八段锦的记录主要是强调外在肢体动作的操作细节，但对其调节人体内在的生理、心理效应及操作方法，并未予以记录。这可能有两个方面的原因，一是八段锦流传时间久、范围广，历史上流派众多，

---

① 八段锦：古人称上等的丝织品为锦，八段锦的名称是将该功法的八节功法比喻为上等的丝织品，以显示其珍贵，称颂其精炼完美的排练和良好的祛病保健作用。
② 湿气：阴暗潮湿的环境或体内的代谢废物。

外在操作形式呈现多样化，内在操作被各流派隐秘起来不被流传；二是内在操作较外在操作的难度更大，对练习者而言掌握较为困难，非文字可以表述清楚。

有鉴于此，在梳理古代八段锦传承文献的基础上，著者结合多年来的教学、科研和临床经验，整理出本套用于养生及针对脊椎病、糖尿病、高血压等慢性病预防、康复的八段锦功法。该功法按照调身、调息、调心三个部分的顺序安排，以便于练习者以此顺序渐次地训练，也就是说，八段锦动作姿势的习练（调身）熟练掌握后，再进入调息训练，而调息训练熟练后才能进入调心的训练。因此，我们建议大家在阅读和训练八段锦时，请按照章节顺序进行习读和训练。

本书英译部分是沈艺教授主持的"北京中医药大学《中医气功学导论》慕课字幕翻译"项目研究成果的进一步升华成果，并得到该项目一定的出版资助。沈艺教授和张晓枚副教授作为本书英文主译，还要由衷感谢方廷钰教授给予英文翻译的指导。同时，感谢胡庆川、李航宇、王莹、郭佳美、张春晓、王婷婷、于雅丽等诸位研究生分别参与中文编辑、慕课字幕英译；由衷感谢程昱博老师对配图的拍摄、编辑等给予的无私帮助和支持。

希望"中医养生功法系列丛书"《八段锦》（汉英对照）有助于传统养生功法的国际推广，服务于全球喜爱中国传统文化和中国功夫的朋友们，以带给大家健康、快乐、和美的生活。

本书不足之处请读者提出宝贵意见，以便再版时修订提高。

魏玉龙

2020年8月19日

Preface

Ba Duan Jin[1] (An Eight-routine Invaluable Qigong Exercise) is currently one of the most popular and effective ancient Chinese Qigong exercises for life nurturing and rehabilitation internationally. It's known as its smooth and elegant movements, especially with a focus on the human spine and the practice techniques of keeping the left-right symmetry, the front-back harmony and the up-down coordination. Through the continuous and overall training of the body, it can promote the circulation of qi and blood throughout the body, strengthen the body and thus achieve the purpose of life nurturing and rehabilitation.

Ba Duan Jin, with a long history and far-reaching inheritance, has its practice method and concept about life nurturing traced back to the Yao and Shun Period in ancient times when the ancestors of the tribe stretched their limbs for training to prevent and treat "dampness[2]". Many of its movements can be found in the illustrated Daoyin in the Han Dynasty and the initial formation of its movements is recorded in *Records of Cultivating Life and Prolonging Life* (Yǎng Xìng Yán Mìng Lù, 养性延命录) written by Tao Hongjing (456-536 A.D.) in the Liang Dynasty of the Southern Dynasties. The name "Ba Duan Jin" was first found in *The Records by Yi Jian* (Yí Jiān Zhì, 夷坚志) written by Hong Mai (1123-1202 A.D.) in the Southern Song Dynasty, while the earliest written record of the whole set of routines can be seen in *The Pivot*

---

① Ba Duan Jin (八段锦 bā duàn jǐn): The finest silk was called brocade in ancient China. As the name of Ba Duan Jin (An Eight-routine Invaluable Qigong Exercise) suggests, the eight-routine exercise is compared to the finest silk, which intends to show its preciousness and praise it for its refined design and good effects of preventing and curing diseases. It's also literally translated as Eight Pieces of Brocade.

② dampness (湿气 shī qì): The dark humidity of the environment and the metabolic wastes in the body. In TCM, it refers to (1) dampness as a pathogenic factor; (2) disease caused by dampness.

of the Dao· Magic Qigong Methods (Dào Shū·Zhòng Miào Piān, 道枢·众妙篇) written by Zeng Zao in the Southern Song Dynasty. The current popular eight routines in verse were first found in *Tips for Ling Jianzi's Daoyin at Noon (Zi) and Midnight (Wu)* (Líng Jiàn Zǐ Dǎo Yǐn Zǐ Wǔ Jué, 灵剑子导引子午诀) in the Song and Yuan Dynasties. Until the end of Ming and early Qing Dynasties, the designations of the routines in Ba Duan Jin were basically finalized and are still in use even nowadays. It's described in verse as "holding both hands high with palms up to regulate the triple energizer, posing as if drawing a bow both left and right to shoot, holding one arm aloft alternately to regulate the functions of the spleen and stomach, looking backward to relieve five consumptions and seven impairments, swinging the head and lowering the body to eliminate stress-induced heart fire, moving the hands down and touching the feet to strengthen the kidney and waist, thrusting the clenched fists forward with glaring eyes to enhance strength, raising and lowering the heels seven times to cure various diseases".

Ba Duan Jin falls into the category of ancient traditional Chinese exercises which include three component parts: the body adjustment (the training of postures), the breath adjustment (the training of breaths) and the mind adjustment (the training of mental states). The documental records of Ba Duan Jin throughout all the previous dynasties mainly emphasized the detailed practice of the external body movements, but no records were found about the physiological and psychological effects induced by its training and regulation or its practice methods. There are two reasons that may account for it. For one reason, there were many schools of Ba Duan Jin in history due to its wide spread and long history. The external body movements were diversified while the practice methods of the internal movements were kept secret by various schools from being spread. For another reason, as compared with the external movements, the internal movements were more difficult for practitioners to master and it's beyond words to express clearly.

Given all this, the author of this book, combined with years of his teaching, scientific research and clinical experiences, has sorted out the Qigong exercises of Ba Duan Jin for the prevention, control, rehabilitation and life nurturing of chronic diseases such as spondylosis, diabetes mellitus and hypertension on the basis of the literary documents and inheritance of ancient Ba Duan Jin. This set of Qigong exercises is arranged according to the order of the body adjustment, the breath adjustment and the mind adjustment so that practitioners can gradually practice in sequence. That is to say, only when you are proficient in the body adjustment of Ba Duan Jin can you proceed to do the practice of the breath adjustment and finally do the practice of the mind adjustment after you become versed in the breath adjustment. Therefore, we recommend that you should follow the chapters of this book in sequence when you read and practice Ba Duan Jin.

The English translation of this book is the fruit of the research on the MOOC subtitle translation project on *Introduction to Chinese Medical Qigong* headed by Professor Shen Yi at Beijing University of Chinese Medicine, which has partly funded the book for its publication. As chief English translators of this book, Professor Shen Yi and Associate Professor Zhang Xiaomei would like to express their sincere appreciation to Professor Fang Tingyu for his good and instructive advice on English translation. At the same time, our sincere gratitude also goes to the postgraduate students Hu Qingchuan, Li Hangyu, Wang Ying and Guo Jiamei for their help with the Chinese editing and Zhang Chunxiao, Wang Tingting and Yu Yali for their active participation in the MOOC subtitle translation. Moreover, we are extremely grateful to Mr. Cheng Yubo for his generous help and support in taking and editing the photos for the illustrations in the book.

We hope *Chinese Medical Qigong Exercises for Nurturing Life* (*Chinese-English Edition*): *Ba Duan Jin* will facilitate the international promotion of this kind of traditional Qigong exercises for nurturing life, serve the friends who love traditional Chinese culture and Chinese Kung Fu all over the world and bring all a healthy, happy and wonderful life.

We'd welcome your valuable comments or suggestions on the book to help us to inprove the revised edition when it's reprinted. Your helpful advice is greatly appreciated.

Wei Yulong

August 19, 2020

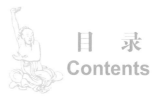

目　录
Contents

第一章　八段锦调身操作

预 备 式

身体呈中正站立位；两脚足跟并拢，足尖外分，使两足的足尖夹角呈45°；膝关节和髋关节要放松，但不要屈曲，臀部回收，小腹部微微内收，腰骶部放松，使腰椎的正常生理曲度得到恢复；胸部不要前挺，微微向内含，同时将背部向上拔伸，注意用意不用力；颈项部肌肉放松，使头部保持中正，不歪斜，调整的技巧是双目平视正前方，以我们的视平面与地面平行为度，目光尽量望向远方；牙齿轻合，嘴唇轻闭，面部肌肉放松，面带微笑，但笑不露齿，做到似笑非笑，以面部不紧张为度；双臂自然放松，置于身体两侧，虚腋（也就是腋窝不可内夹，要留有大约自己一个拳头的空间）、松肩（也就是肩关节既不能向上耸起，也不能向内下方夹紧，保持一个肩关节整体放松状态），肘关节和腕关节微微弯曲，以能够自然放松为度，整个手掌放松，掌心向内，五指微曲（图1-0-1、图1-0-2）。

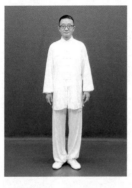 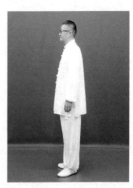

图1-0-1 (Fig.1-0-1)　　　　　　图1-0-2 (Fig.1-0-2)

Chapter 1 Body Adjustment Practice of Ba Duan Jin

Preparatory Posture

Stand with the body in a centered and upright position. Keep heels together and tiptoes apart at a 45-degree angle. Relax the knee and hip joints, never bend them, with the buttocks in and the lower abdomen slightly adducted. Loosen up the lumbosacral part to restore the normal physiological curvature of the lumbar spine. Do not have the chest raised up, but slightly adducted with the back extending up simultaneously. Remember to do it with the guided mind rather than the strength. Keep the neck muscles relaxed and the head in a centered rather than skewed position. The tip for the adjustment is to look straight ahead, parallel to the ground and look as far away as possible. Close the teeth and lips slightly. Relax the facial muscles. Hold a smile on the face. Smile without showing the teeth. Keep a faint smile without any facial tension. Relax the arms and place them on both sides of the body naturally. Loosen up the armpits (Armpits should not be clamped in and there should be one fist-width space left.) and relax the shoulders (Shoulders can neither be raised upward nor held tightly inward and downward. Keep them relaxed.). Slightly bend the elbows and wrists in a naturally relaxing way. Keep the entire palms relaxed with palms inward and fingers slightly bent. (Fig.1-0-1, Fig.1-0-2)

第一节　两手托天理三焦

1. 调身训练步骤

（1）预备式（图1-1-1、图1-1-2）

两足的足跟并拢，脚尖向外分开成45°。双手自然垂在身体的两侧，目光平视远方。意识收回体内，全身自然放松。

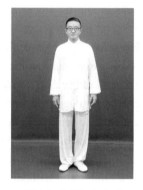　　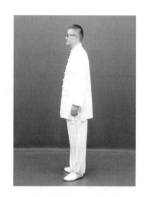

图1-1-1 (Fig.1-1-1)　　　　图1-1-2 (Fig.1-1-2)

（2）体侧提掌（图1-1-3、图1-1-4）

首先，两腕关节微曲，掌心向后，指尖向下，两手沿体侧的足少阳胆经，缓缓地提起，至两侧髂棘高度，两肘关节内收，肩关节下沉，全身放松。

Routine 1 Holding Both Hands High with Palms Up to Regulate the Triple Energizer

1. Step−by−step Instructions

(1) Preparatory posture (Fig.1-1-1, Fig.1-1-2)

Stand with heels together and tiptoes apart at a 45-degree angle. Place both hands naturally alongside the body. Look straight ahead. Keep the whole body relaxed naturally with the concentration of the mind on the internal body.

(2) Lifting the palms from both sides of the body (Fig.1-1-3, Fig.1-1-4)

First, keep wrists slightly bent, palms backward and fingertips downward. Lift both hands slowly to the iliac crest level along the Gall-bladder Meridian of Foot-*Shaoyang* on both sides of the body. Keep the elbows adducted, the shoulders relaxed and the whole body loosened up.

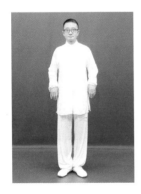 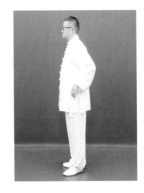

图1−1−3 (Fig.1−1−3)　　图1−1−4 (Fig.1−1−4)

（3）托天提踵（图1-1-5～图1-1-9）

双掌向外翻掌，使掌心向上，手如托物，缓缓自体侧向体前上托，托至肩关节的高度。

两掌在肩关节的水平，以腕关节为轴，缓缓向前、前外、外、外后、内进行旋转，当旋转至外后时，两肘关节顺势外撑，使双手指尖相对，掌心保持向上，不可偏斜。

双手继续沿耳郭两侧，缓缓上托，与此同时，膝关节挺直，两腿内后侧（足少阴肾经[①]）微微夹紧，微微抬（慢慢提）起两侧足跟，使其缓缓离开地面（注意不宜太高，仅以不接触地面为度），足趾抓紧地面，头部引领整个身体，微微向后上方伸展。

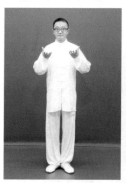
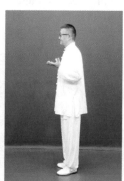
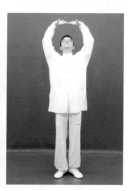

图1-1-5 (Fig.1-1-5)　　　图1-1-6 (Fig.1-1-6)　　　图1-1-7 (Fig.1-1-7)

---

① 足少阴肾经：起于足小趾之下，斜过足心，出于舟骨粗隆下，沿内踝之后，进入足跟中，向上行于小腿内侧，出腘窝内侧，上行大腿内侧后缘，穿过脊柱，属于肾，络于膀胱。其主干，从肾上穿肝、膈，进入肺中，沿着喉咙，夹舌根旁。其支脉，从肺出来，络于心，注于胸中。

(3) Pushing hands skyward and raising heels off the ground (Fig.1-1-5～Fig.1-1-9)

Rotate both hands outward so that the palms face upward. Raise up the hands slowly along both sides of the body toward the front of the body and push them skyward as if lifting an object to the shoulder level.

At the shoulder level, slowly rotate both palms forward, outward, backward and inward with the wrist as an axis. When rotating the palms outward and backward, stretch the elbows outward with fingertips facing each other and palms up without any slant.

Continue to hold up the hands along the auricles on both sides slowly, at the same time, keep the knees straight and the inner back of the legs (Kidney Meridian of Foot-*Shaoyin*[1]) slightly clamped. Slightly raise the heels to be off the ground slowly (not too high, just to the extent of not touching the ground). Clutch the ground with the toes and direct the whole body to stretch backward and upward slightly with the head.

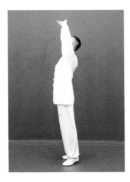 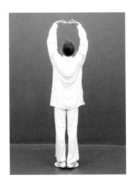

图1-1-8 (Fig.1-1-8)　　图1-1-9 (Fig.1-1-9)

[1] Kidney Meridian of Foot-*Shaoyin*: Kidney Meridian of Foot-*Shaoyin* starts from the interior side of the little toe and runs obliquely toward the sole. Emerging from below the tuberosity of navicular bone and running behind the medial malleolus, it enters the heel. From there, it rises along the medial side of the leg to the medial side of the popliteal fossa, goes up along the posteromedial side of the thigh toward the vertebral column where it enters the kidney that it pertains to and connects with the bladder. Its main meridian ascends and passes through the liver and diaphragm from above the kidneys. Then it enters the lungs, runs along the throat and is clamped at the root of the tongue. Its branch comes from the lungs, connects with the heart and runs into the chest.

当双手托至头顶，让双手的中指指尖（中冲穴①）相接，头部继续向后上方伸展，目视双掌之间，继续向上托举，以双掌平面与地面平行为度，两臂不可挺直，使双臂、双掌围拢成圆，中指尖与肚脐（神阙穴②）的连线与地面保持垂直。

保持此托天伸展的状态，停顿1个呼吸的时间（约5秒）。

（4）手足同落

然后，两中指分开，两臂缓缓分别沿身体两侧外展下落，头部引领整个身体，慢慢恢复到中正的状态，双目平视正前方，同时足跟缓缓落地，双足踏实地面。恢复到预备式。

2. 易犯错误

（1）足跟不能并拢，膝关节屈曲，致使下肢内后侧的足少阴肾经不能受到刺激，力量被分解，不能够一气贯通向上直达颠顶。

（2）托天提踵时，出现耸肩、夹肩，致使手三阳经③和手三阴经④的气血在肩部阻滞不通，造成肩背部连及颈项部肌群紧张，气血不通，引起头晕、心悸等症状。

（3）头部塌缩或头颈部位置不中正，造成颈项部紧张和左右不平衡，致使头颈部左右、前后的气血分布不均衡。

---

① 中冲穴：属于手厥阴心包经的穴位，位于中指末端的最高点。
② 神阙穴：属于任脉的穴位，位于脐区，肚脐的中央。
③ 手三阳经：是手阳明大肠经、手太阳小肠经、手少阳三焦经三条经脉的合称。
④ 手三阴经：是手太阴肺经、手少阴心经、手厥阴心包经三条经脉的合称。

When holding up the hands over the top of the head, let the middle fingertips of the hands (Zhongchong[1]) connect and stretch the head backward and upward with the eyes gazing at the back of palms. Then, continue to hold up the hands to keep the palms parallel to the ground. Don't stretch the arms straight. Instead, bring the arms and palms together to form a circle with the linking line between the middle fingertips and the navel (Shenque[2]) perpendicular to the ground.

Hold this position of stretching and pushing the hands skyward with palms up and pause for one breath (about five seconds).

(4) Putting down the hands and heels at the same time

Then, keep the two middle fingers apart and the arms slowly down along both sides of the body. The whole body is directed by the head slowly to return to the center. Look straight ahead with the heels slowly down to the ground and the feet firmly on the ground. Return to the preparatory posture.

2. Common Mistakes

(1) The heels are not closed together and the knees are bent. As a result, the Kidney Meridian of Foot-*Shaoyin* at the internal back sides of the lower limbs cannot be stimulated, which makes the strength decomposed and fail to reach the top of the head.

(2) Shrug and clamp the shoulders in the movement of pushing hands skyward and raising heels off the ground, which causes the qi and blood of the three yang meridians of the hand[3] and the three yin meridians of the hand[4] to be blocked at the shoulders. Consequently, the muscles of shoulders, back and neck become tense, which induces a blockage of the circulation of qi and blood. Then such symptoms as dizziness, palpitations and so on may ensue.

(3) The head droops down or the head and neck are not kept in a centered and upright position, which results in a neck tension, a left and right imbalance and an uneven distribution of qi and blood all around the head and neck.

---

[1] Zhongchong (PC9): an acupoint of the Pericardium Meridian of Hand-*Jueyin*, at the tip of the middle finger
[2] Shenque (CV8): an acupoint of the Conception Vessel, at the center of the navel region
[3] three yang meridians of the hand: a collective term for the Large Intestine Meridian of Hand-*Yangming*, the Small Intestine Meridian of Hand-*Taiyang* and the Triple Energizer Meridian of Hand-*Shaoyang*
[4] three yin meridians of the hand: a collective term for the Lung Meridian of Hand-*Taiyin*, the Heart Meridian of Hand-*Shaoyin* and the Pericardium Meridian of Hand-*Jueyin*

（4）两掌松弛无力，则不能通过腕关节带动肘关节、肩关节协同运动，致使手三阳经和手三阴经得不到螺旋式牵拉，不能有效调动手部经气运转和畅达。

3. 操作强度

如果本节功法与全套功法一起操作，一般情况操作3次或6次。

如果单独操作本节功法，可以根据自身状况，按照3、6、9、12的次数递增运动量，直至身体微微汗出为度。

4. 功法作用

三焦为六腑之一，是上、中、下三焦的合称。关于"焦"字的含义，历代医家认识不一。有认为"焦"当作"膲"（jiāo）者，膲为体内脏器，是有形之物；有认为"焦"字从火，为无形之气，能腐熟水谷；有认为"焦"字当作"樵"（qiáo）字，樵，槌也，节也，谓人体上、中、下三节段或三个区域。三焦，作为六腑之一，位于躯体和脏腑之间的空腔，包含胸腔和腹腔，人体的其他脏腑器官均在其中，即将躯干划分为3个部位，横膈以上内脏器官为上焦，包括心、肺；横膈以下至脐为中焦，包括脾、胃、肝、胆等内脏（肝，按其部位来说，应划归中焦，但因它与肾关系密切，故将肝和肾一同划归下焦）；脐以下为下焦，包括肾、大肠、小肠、膀胱。所以六腑当中，唯三焦最大，无与匹配，故有"孤府"之称。正如张景岳所说："三焦者，确有一腑，盖脏腑之外，躯壳之内，包罗诸脏，一腔之大腑也。"（《类经·藏象类》）。

(4) The two palms are flabby and weak so that the elbows and shoulders cannot collaborate to move through the wrist joints. As a result, the three yang meridians of the hand and the three yin meridians of the hand cannot be spirally stretched, and the qi of the hand meridians fails to be effectively mobilized to circulate and flow freely.

3. Amount of Qigong Exercises

This routine, when performed together with a full set of Qigong exercises, is generally done 3 or 6 times.

When doing this routine alone, you can gradually increase the amount of exercise by 3, 6, 9 or 12 times according to your own condition till there is a slight sweat all over the body.

4. Functions and Effects

The triple energizer (Sanjiao), one of the six *fu*-organs, is a collective term for the upper, middle and lower energizers. The word "焦" (jiāo) has been interpreted differently by the medical experts of all dynasties. Some hold that the word "焦" is taken as "膲" (jiāo) which refers to an internal organ and thus it is something visible; some think that the word "焦" pertains to fire and is a kind of invisible qi, which can rot and ripen water and grain; others regard the word "焦" as "樵" (qiáo) which denotes segments, representing the three sections or areas of the human body, i.e. the upper, middle and lower parts of the body. The triple energizer, as one of the six *fu*-organs, is located in the cavity between the trunk and viscera, including the thoracic and abdominal cavities. The other organs of the human body are all inside it, namely, the torso is divided into three parts. The upper energizer covers the area above the diaphragm, including the heart and lungs; the middle energizer extends from below the diaphragm downward to the navel, including the spleen, stomach, liver, gallbladder and other internal organs (Liver, according to its location, should fall into the middle energizer. However, due to its close relationship with the kidneys, it is classified into the lower energizer together with the kidneys). The lower energizer is located below the navel, including the kidneys, large intestine, small intestine and urinary bladder. Therefore, among the six *fu*-organs, the triple energizer is the largest one and has no corresponding *zang*-organ to be paired with. For this reason, it is called a "solitary *fu*-organ". Just as Zhang Jingyue (1563A.D.-1640A.D., a great physician in the Ming Dynasty) said, "The triple energizer is indeed a large *fu*-organ, located outside the *zang-fu* organs but inside the body, covering all the internal organs." (in *The Classified Classic·Visceral Manifestations*) (Lèi Jīng Zàng Xiàng Lèi, 类经 · 藏象类)

三焦具有以下功能：

一是通行元气，首见于《难经》。如《难经·三十一难》说："三焦者，水谷之道路，气之所终始也。"《难经·三十八难》说："所以腑有六者，谓三焦也，有原气之别焉，主持诸气。"《难经·六十六难》说："三焦者，原气之别使也，主通行三气，经历于五脏六腑。"原文明确地说明三焦是人体元气（原气）升降出入的道路，人体元气是通过三焦而到达五脏六腑和全身各处的。元气，为人体最根本的气，是生命活动的原动力。元气根于肾，通过三焦别入十二经脉而达于五脏六腑，故称三焦为元气之别使。《中藏经·论三焦虚实寒热生死逆顺脉证之法》对三焦通行元气的生理作用做了更为具体的描述："三焦者，人之三元之气也，号曰中清之府，总领五脏六腑、营卫、经络、内外、左右、上下之气也。三焦通，则内外左右上下皆通也，其于周身灌体，和内调外，营左养右，导上宣下，莫大于此也。"因为三焦通行元气于全身，是人体之气升降出入的通道，亦是气化的场所，故称三焦有主持诸气，总司全身气机和气化的功能。如果元气虚弱，三焦通道运行不畅或衰退，就会导致全身或某些部位的气虚现象。

The triple energizer has the following functions:

Firstly, the triple energizer transports and moves the original qi, firstly seen in *The Classic of Difficult Issues* (Nàn Jīng, 难经). For instance, in *The Classic of Difficult Issues · Thirty-first Difficult Issue*, it says: "The triple energizer encompasses the passageways of water and grain. It represents the ending and the beginning of the course of qi." In *The Classic of Difficult Issues · Thirty-eighth Difficult Issue*, it states, "The triple energizer is to be named as the reason for the fact that there are six *fu*-organs. The triple energizer represents an additional source of original qi; it governs all the qi circulating in the body." In *The Classic of Difficult Issue · Sixty-sixth Difficult Issues*, it says, "The triple energizer is the special envoy that transmits the original qi. It is responsible for the passage of the three qi through the five *zang*-organs and six *fu*-organs." The original text clearly expounds that the triple energizer is the passageway of the original qi in the body to ascend and descend, exit and enter. It is through the triple energizer that the original qi of the body can reach the *zang-fu* organs and the whole body. The original qi, as the most fundamental qi of the human body, is a motive force of life activities. It has its root in the kidneys. It enters the twelve meridians through the triple energizer and reaches the five *zang*-organs and six *fu*-organs. For this reason, the triple energizer is considered as the special envoy that transmits the original qi. In *The Treasured Classic ·Treatise on Pulses and Patterns of Deficiency and Excess, Cold and Heat, Life and Death, Abnormality and Normality in the Triple Energizer* (Zhōng Zàng Jīng· Lùn Sān Jiāo Xū Shí Hán Rè Shēng Sǐ Nì Shùn Mài Zhèng Zhī Fǎ, 中藏经 · 论三焦虚实寒热生死逆顺脉证之法), there is a detailed description on the physiological functions of the triple energizer : "The triple energizer is responsible for the passage of the triple original qi of the body. It is called the *fu*-organ of clarity and purity. The triple energizer is in charge of the qi of the five *zang*-organs and six *fu*-organs, nutritive and defensive qi, the qi of meridians and collaterals, internal and external qi, left and right qi, upward and downward qi. If the triple energizer is free of blockage, so are the rest parts of the body. The triple energizer can be infused into the whole body and utilized to harmonize the interior and exterior of the body, nourish the left and right, guide the upward and diffuse the downward. And nothing else is more precious than this". As it transmits the original qi all through the body and serves as the passageway of the upward, downward, outward and inward movements of qi as well as an arena for qi transformation, the triple energizer governs all the qi circulating in the body and the functions of qi movement and transformation. If the original qi is weak or the triple energizer is blocked or declined, it may lead to qi deficiency of the whole body or in some parts of the body.

二是运行水谷，《素问·五脏别论》称三焦为传化之腑，其具有传化水谷的功能。《素问·六节藏象论》说："三焦……仓廪之本，营之居也，名曰器，能化糟粕，转味而入出者也。"指出三焦具有将水谷精微变化为营气，以及传化糟粕的作用。《难经》明确提出三焦运行水谷的作用，如《难经·三十一难》说："三焦者，水谷之道路，气之所终始也。上焦者，在心下，下膈，在胃上口，主内而不出……中焦者，在胃中脘，不上不下，主腐熟水谷……下焦者，当膀胱上口，主分别清浊，主出而不内。"水谷在人体的运行道路及气之所终始，包括饮食物的消化、精微物质的吸收、糟粕的排泄全部过程，用"三焦者，水谷之道路"来概括。并因上、中、下三焦所处部位不同，对水谷运行过程中所起的作用也就不同，而有上焦主纳，中焦主腐熟，下焦主分别清浊、主出的具体描述。这是以三焦运行水谷来概括饮食物的消化、吸收及排泄的功能。

Secondly, the triple energizer transports and transforms water and food. In *Plain Questions· Different Discussion on the Five Zang-Organs* [9] (Sù Wèn ·Wǔ Zàng Bié Lùn, 素问 · 五脏别论), the triple energizer is called the *fu*-organ of transmission and transformation, which functions as transporting and transforming water and food. In *Plain Questions· Discussion on Six-Plus-Six System and the Manifestations of the Viscera* (Sù Wèn · Liù Jié Zàng Xiàng Lùn, 素问 · 六节藏象论) , it says, "… the triple energizer… are the roots of granary and the location of nutrient qi. These organs are called containers because they can store food, transform waste materials and manage the transformation, absorption and discharge of the flavors." It points out that the triple energizer can turn food essence into nutrient qi and function as transporting and transforming waste substances in the body. *The Classic of Difficult Issues* (Nàn Jīng, 难经) clearly puts forward that the triple energizer has the function of transporting water and food. For instance, *The Classic of Difficult Issues · Thirty-first Difficult Issue* says, "The triple energizer encompasses the passageways of water and grain. It represents the ending and the beginning of the course of the qi. The upper energizer extends from below the heart downward through the diaphragm and ends at the upper opening of the stomach. It is responsible for intake but not for discharge ... The middle energizer is located in the middle stomach cavity; it doesn't extend further upward or downward. It is responsible for the spoiling and processing of water and grain ... The lower energizer begins exactly at the upper opening of the urinary bladder and extends downward. It is responsible for separating the clear from the turbid portions. It contains discharge but not intake." The circulating route of water and grain in the body, the ending and the beginning of the course of qi and the whole process of the digestion of water and food, the absorption of food essence and the discharge of the waste can be summarized as " The triple energizer encompasses the passageways of water and grain." As the upper, middle and lower energizers are located differently, they play different roles in the process of transporting and transforming water and food. The upper energizer is in charge of food intake, the middle energizer is in charge of spoiling and processing food and grains, the lower energizer is responsible for separating the clear from the turbid portions and in charge of excretion as well. It summarizes the digestion, absorption and excretion of water and food from the perspective of the triple energizer in the transportation and transformation of water and food.

三是运行水液，三焦为人体水液运行的主要通道，这在《黄帝内经》中有多处论述，如《素问·灵兰秘典论》说："三焦者，决渎之官，水道出焉。"《灵枢·本输》说："三焦者，中渎之腑，水道出焉，属膀胱，是孤之腑也。"说明三焦是人体管理水液的器官，有疏通水道，运行水液的作用。人体水液代谢是一个复杂的生理过程，是多个脏腑的一系列生理功能的综合作用。如《素问·经脉别论》说："饮入于胃，游溢精气，上输于脾，脾气散精，上归于肺，通调水道，下输膀胱，水精四布，五经并行。"水液代谢虽由胃、脾、肺、肾、肠、膀胱等脏腑共同协作而完成，但人体水液的升降出入，周身环流，则必须以三焦为通道才能实现。因此，三焦水道的通利与否，不仅影响水液运行的迟速，而且也必然影响有关脏腑对水液的输布与排泄功能。也可以说，三焦运行水液，是对脾、肺、肾等脏腑主管水液代谢作用的综合概括。如果三焦水道不利，则脾、肺、肾等脏腑调节水液的功能将难以实现，引起水液代谢的失常，水液输布与排泄障碍，产生痰饮、水肿等病变。正如《类经·藏象类》所说："上焦不治，则水泛高原；中焦不治，则水留中脘；下焦不治，则水乱二便。"

Thirdly, the triple energizer transports and moves water and body fluids. The triple energizer is the major passageway for the movement of the body fluids, which has frequently been documented in *Huang-di's Canon of Medicine* (Huáng Di Nèi Jīng, 黄帝内经). For instance, *Plain Questions· Discussion on the Secret Canons Stored in Royal Library* (Sù Wèn · Líng Lán Mì Diǎn Lùn, 素问 · 灵兰秘典论) states, " The triple energizer is the organ similar to official in charge of dredging and is responsible for regulating the water passage." *Spiritual Pivot · Discussion on Acupoints* (Líng Shū ·Běn Shū, 灵枢 · 本输) says, " The triple energizer is a water-regulating *fu*-organ which guides water passage, pertains to the urinary bladder and is a solitary *fu*-organ." This statement shows that the triple energizer is an organ that regulates the water and body fluids in the body, functioning as dredging water channels and moving water and body fluids. Water metabolism of the human body is a complex physiological process, which is completed by the cooperation of many organs. Just as *Plain Questions· Special Discussion on the Channels and Vessels* (Sù Wèn ·Jīng Mài Bié Lù, 素问 · 经脉别论) states, "When water is taken into the stomach, the essence-qi is distributed around and transported to the spleen. The spleen qi spreads the essence and transports it upward to the lung which regulates water channel and transports water downward to the urinary bladder. In this way, the essence of water is distributed all through the body and into the five channels simultaneously." Although the metabolism of water and fluids is completed through the coordinated work of the stomach, spleen, lungs, kidneys, intestines, bladder and other organs, it is through the triple energizer channel that the upward, downward, outward and inward movements of the body fluids and their circulation in the whole body can be realized. Therefore, whether the triple energizer channel is free of blockage or not will not only affect the speed of water movement, but also affect the water distribution and excretion of relevant *zang-fu* organs. It can be said that the triple energizer moving water and body fluids gives a comprehensive summary to the functions of the spleen, lungs, kidneys in charge of water metabolism. If the water channel of the triple energizer is blocked, it is difficult for the spleen, lungs, kidneys to perform the function of regulating water and body fluids, which may result in abnormal water metabolism, disorder of water distribution and excretion, causing phlegm and edema. Just as *The Classified Classic·Visceral Manifestations* (Lèi Jīng·Zàng Xiàng Lèi, 类经 · 藏象类) says, "If the upper triple energizer is out of control, the water will flood the plateau (to cause the functional disorder of the heart and lungs). If the middle triple energizer is out of control, the water will be blocked in the middle stomach cavity (to cause the functional disorder of the stomach and spleen). If the lower triple energizer is out of control, the blocked water will cause the functional disorder of the urinary bladder and intestines."

本节功法表面看是两手托举、足跟离地的动作操作，实则是以意识诱导存想托举重物，头部为动作的主要引导方向，同时五个脚趾紧抓地面，协调向上，缓缓用力，纵向牵拉、伸展全身各部软组织（人体绝大部分经脉是纵向分布的），拉宽椎间隙，对防治颈部、肩部、腰部疾患有良好的效果。上托时的旋掌动作，对于提高腕关节、肘关节、肩关节灵活性和柔韧度有一定康复作用。

第二节　左右开弓似射雕

本节功法分左式和右式两式，按照先左后右的顺序，左右两式交替进行操作。

1. 调身训练步骤

（1）预备式（图1-2-1、图1-2-2）

两足跟并拢，足尖外分。两手自然垂在身体两侧，目视远方，全身放松。

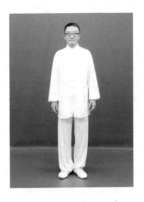 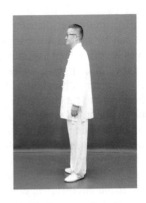

图1-2-1 (Fig.1-2-1)　　　　图1-2-2 (Fig.1-2-2)

This routine appears to be a practice of holding both hands high with palms up and heels off the ground. In fact, it is a practice of inducing inward contemplation of lifting a heavy object guided by the mind and taking the head as the main guiding part to pull the whole body upward. At the same time, with the five toes clutched to the ground, the soft tissues of every part of the whole body are longitudinally pulled and stretched (for most meridians of the human body distributed longitudinally) with a coordinated, upward and slow force. Pulling the intervertebral spaces wide has a good effect on treating the neck, shoulder and waist diseases. The movement of rotating palms when holding the hands high can improve the flexibility and softness of the wrists, elbows and shoulders in the rehabilitation.

Routine 2   Posing as if Drawing a Bow Both Left and Right to Shoot

This routine includes the left and right postures. Start with left first and then right. Both are practiced alternately in sequence.

1. Step-by-step Instructions

(1) Preparatory posture (Fig.1-2-1, Fig.1-2-2)

Stand with heels together and tiptoes apart. Place both hands naturally alongside the body. Look straight ahead. Keep the whole body relaxed.

（2）左式开步（图1-2-3）

左脚向左前方45°方向，迈出一大步，步宽为自身肩宽的1.5倍左右，左脚尖微微内扣，使两脚内侧面平行，上身仍面向正前方，双目平视正前方。

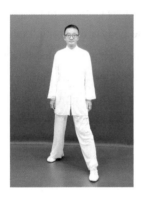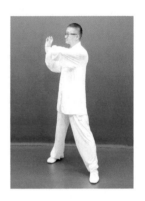

图1-2-3 (Fig.1-2-3)　　图1-2-4 (Fig.1-2-4)

（3）转身错掌（图1-2-4）

上身缓缓向右旋转，旋转至上身与两腿在同一平面时，肩关节、肘关节、腕关节放松微曲，如鸟的翅膀一样，自身体两侧缓缓地抬起，抬至腕关节与肩关节同高。此时，肘关节下沉，应略低于肩关节与腕关节的水平。

然后，两掌沿肩关节水平缓缓内收，至胸前两腕关节靠拢交叉，左手在前，右手在后。左手五指微屈，大拇指在外，握于其余四指末端指关节的背侧，握成空拳。右手五指屈曲，大拇指与其余四指相对成"爪"状。

（4）下蹲开弓（图1-2-5、图1-2-6）

两脚同时屈膝，慢慢下蹲成马步，身体保持中正，垂直下蹲，躯干不可向前俯，也不可向后仰，膝关节的屈曲程度需根据自身情况酌定，一般保持在90°～150°范围即可。

蹲稳马步后，上身微微向左平移，将重心移至左腿，使左膝关节的屈曲程度大于右膝关节，两脚踏实地面。

在重心移到左腿的同时，左手空拳沿肩部平面向左拉至肩关节的前部，距离肩关节一拳的距离。

(2) Starting with the left foot (Fig.1-2-3)

Take a big step with the left foot toward a 45-degree direction in the left front. The step is about 1.5 times as wide as the shoulders. Clutch the ground with the left tiptoes slightly in to keep the inner sides of the feet parallel to each other. The upper body still faces right ahead. Look straight ahead.

(3) Turning around and crossing the palms (Fig.1-2-4)

Rotate the upper body slowly to the right till it is aligned with the legs. At the same time, keep the shoulders, elbows and wrists relaxed and slightly bent. Like a bird flapping its wings, raise the arms slowly from both sides of the body until the wrists reach the shoulder level. Meanwhile, keep the elbows down slightly below the level of shoulders and wrists.

Then, slowly adduct both palms along the shoulder level to the front of the chest, where the two wrists are brought close and crossed, with the left hand in front of the right one. Slightly bend the five fingers of the left hand with the thumb outward. Hold the thumb on the back of the end knuckles of the other four fingers to make a hollow fist. Bend the five fingers of the right hand with the thumb facing the other four fingers to form a claw-like position.

(4) Squatting and posing as if drawing a bow (Fig.1-2-5, Fig.1-2-6)

Bend the knees of both legs simultaneously, squat down slowly into a horse stance, keep the body in a centered position and a vertical squatting posture. Don't lean the torso forward or backward. Keep the knees bent in a range of $90° \sim 150°$ according to your own situation.

With a steady horse stance, move the upper body slowly to the left by shifting the body weight to the left leg. The left knee is bent greater than the right knee with both feet firmly anchored on the ground.

While shifting the body weight to the left leg, pull the left hollow fist horizontally along the shoulder to the front of the shoulder joint, one fist-width away from it.

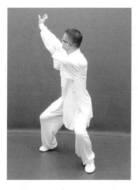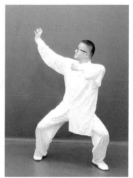

图1-2-5 (Fig.1-2-5)　　　图1-2-6 (Fig.1-2-6)

右手腕关节背屈，掌心向右，缓缓向右上方推出，推至右耳郭的高度。两手对抗用力，如开弓射箭状。

在双手对抗拉弓的同时，上身向左倾斜10°～15°，随着向上方推弓，双目通过右手虎口^①，如瞄准前上方飞翔的大雕，伺机射出。

保持射雕的姿势，停顿1个呼吸的时间（注意可默念1至5个数字，也可做1个腹式呼吸运动以度量时间）。

（5）起身合掌（图1-2-7）

两臂缓缓松力，两手缓缓向胸前正中线回撤，合掌置于胸前。

与此同步，将身体重心慢慢移至两腿中间，恢复到马步姿势，缓缓起身。

然后，两掌沿胸前中线缓缓下落，落至肚脐水平，两掌自然分开，分置于大腿两侧。

与此同步，上身缓缓向左磨转，恢复到上身面向正前方的状态。左脚收回，恢复到预备式的站立位。

① 虎口：手掌背侧第一、二掌骨之间的区域。

Bend the right wrist backward with the palm facing right and slowly push it upward to the height of the right auricle. Pull with both hands oppositely as if drawing a bow to shoot an arrow.

While drawing the bow with both hands as if drawing a bow to shoot, tilt the upper body left to $10°\sim15°$. As the bow is pushed upward, look through Hukou[①] of the right hand, as if aiming at a big eagle flying overhead in the front and waiting for an opportunity to shoot.

Hold this position of shooting an eagle and pause for one breath (counting silently from 1 to 5 or taking one abdominal breath to measure time).

(5) Rising to your feet and putting the palms together (Fig.1-2-7)

Relax the two arms gradually, adduct both hands slowly toward the midline of the chest and put the palms together in front of the chest.

Simultaneously, shift the body weight slowly to the middle of the legs, return to the horse stance and rise to your feet slowly.

Then, put down both palms slowly along the midline of the chest to the navel level. Separate the two palms naturally and place them at both sides of the thighs.

At the same time, swing the upper body to the left slowly and return to the position of the upper body facing straight ahead. Retract the left foot and return to the preparatory standing posture.

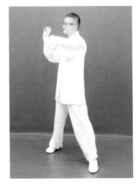

图1-2-7 (Fig.1-2-7)

① Hukou (虎口 hǔ kǒu): area between the first and second metacarpal bones on the dorsal side of the palm

（6）右式开步（图1-2-8）

右脚向右前方45°方向，迈开一大步，步宽为自身肩宽的1.5倍左右，右脚尖微微内扣，使两脚内侧面平行，上身仍面向正前方，双目平视正前方。

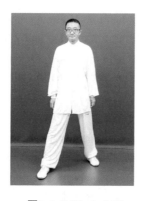 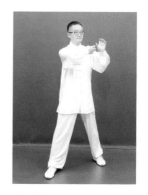

图1-2-8 (Fig.1-2-8)　　　　图1-2-9 (Fig.1-2-9)

（7）转身错掌（图1-2-9）

上身继续向左旋转，旋转至上身与两腿在同一平面；肩关节、肘关节、腕关节放松微曲，如鸟的翅膀一样，自身体两侧缓缓地抬起，抬至腕关节与肩同高时，肘关节下沉，应略低于肩关节与腕关节的水平。

然后，两掌沿肩关节水平缓缓内收，至胸前两腕关节靠拢交叉，右手在前，左手在后。

右手五指微屈，大拇指在外，握于其余四指末端指关节的背侧，握成空拳。左手五指屈曲，大拇指与其余四指相对成"爪"状。

（8）下蹲开弓（图1-2-10）

两腿同时屈膝，慢慢下蹲成马步，身体保持中正，继续下蹲，躯干不可向前俯，也不可向后仰，膝关节的屈曲程度需根据自身情况酌定，一般保持在90°～150°范围即可。

(6) Starting with the right foot (Fig.1-2-8)

Take a big step with your right foot toward a 45-degree direction in the right front. The step is about 1.5 times as wide as the shoulders. Clutch the ground with the right tiptoes slightly in to keep the inner sides of the feet parallel to each other. The upper body still faces right ahead. Look straight ahead.

(7) Turning around and crossing the palms (Fig.1-2-9)

Rotate the upper body slowly to the left till it is aligned with the legs. At the same time, keep the shoulders, elbows, and wrists relaxed and slightly bent. Like a bird flapping its wings, raise the arms slowly from both sides of the body until the wrists reach the shoulder level. Meanwhile, keep the elbows down slightly below the level of shoulders and wrists.

Then, adduct both palms slowly along the shoulder level to the front of the chest, where the two wrists are brought close and crossed, with the right hand in front of the left one.

Slightly bend the five fingers of the right hand with the thumb outward. Hold the thumb on the back of the end knuckles of the other four fingers to make a hollow fist. Bend the five fingers of the left hand with the thumb facing the other four fingers to form a claw-like posture.

(8) Squatting and posing as if drawing a bow (Fig.1-2-10)

Bend the knees of both legs simulta-neously, squat down slowly into a horse stance, keep the body in a centered position and a vertical squatting posture. Don't lean the body forward or backward. Keep the knees bent in a range of 90°～150 ° according to your own situation.

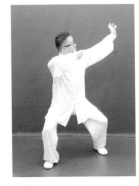

图1-2-10 (Fig.1-2-10)

蹲稳马步后，上身缓缓向右平移，将重心移至右腿，使右膝关节的屈曲程度大于左膝关节，两脚踏实地面。

在重心移到右腿的同时，右手空拳沿肩部平面向右拉至肩关节前部，距离肩关节一拳的距离。

左手腕关节背屈，掌心向左，缓缓向左上方推出，推至左耳郭的高度。两手对抗用力，如开弓射箭状。

在双手对抗拉弓的同时，上身向右倾斜10°～15°，随着向上方推弓，双目通过左手虎口，如瞄准前上方飞翔的大雕，伺机射出。

保持开弓射雕的姿势，停顿1个呼吸的时间（注意可默念1至5个数字，也可做1个腹式呼吸运动以度量时间）。

（9）起身合掌（图1-2-11、图1-2-12）

两臂缓缓松力，两手缓缓向胸前正中线回撤，合掌置于胸前。

与此同时，将身体重心慢慢移至两腿中间，恢复到马步姿势，缓缓起身。

然后，两掌沿胸前中线缓缓下落，落至肚脐水平，两掌自然分开，分置于大腿两侧。

与此同时，上身缓缓向右磨转，恢复到上身面向正前方的状态。

右脚收回，恢复到预备式的站立位。

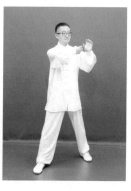 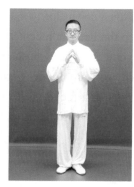

图1-2-11 (Fig.1-2-11)　　　图1-2-12 (Fig.1-2-12)

With a steady horse stance, move the upper body slowly to the right by shifting the body weight to the right leg. The right knee is bent greater than the left knee with both feet firmly anchored on the ground.

While shifting the body weight to the right leg, pull the right hollow fist horizontally along the shoulder to the front of the shoulder joint, one fist-width away from it.

Bend the left wrist backward with the palm facing left and slowly push it upward to the height of the left auricle. Pull with both hands oppositely as if drawing a bow to shoot an arrow.

While drawing the bow with both hands, tilt the upper body right to $10°\sim15°$. As the bow is pushed upward, look through Hukou of the left hand, as if aiming at a big eagle flying overhead in the front and waiting for an opportunity to shoot.

Hold the position of drawing a bow and shooting an eagle and pause for one breath (counting silently from 1 to 5 or taking one abdominal breath to measure time).

(9) Rising to your feet and putting the palms together (Fig.1-2-11, Fig.1-2-12)

Relax the two arms gradually, adduct both hands slowly toward the midline of the chest and put the palms together in front of the chest.

Simultaneously, shift the body weight to the middle of your legs slowly, return to the horse stance and rise to your feet slowly.

Then, put down both palms slowly along the midline of the chest to the navel level. Separate the two palms naturally and place them at both sides of the thighs.

At the same time, swing the upper body to the right slowly and return to the position of the upper body facing straight ahead.

Retract the right foot and return to the preparatory standing posture.

2. 易犯错误

（1）出腿出脚不是在正前方左、右45°角的方向。

（2）出脚后脚尖未能内扣造成两脚不平行（也就是我们日常所说的外八字）。

（3）抬臂时耸肩、塌腰^①；开弓时，两臂没有做到对抗用力，造成胸部前挺，两手虚空无力。

（4）下蹲开弓时，身体的重心没有移到相应的一侧（左式应移动重心到左腿，右式应移动重心到右腿），同时上身没有向相应的一侧微微倾斜（左式应向左倾斜，右式应向右倾斜）。

（5）起身合掌时，未能将重心移回身体中线就直接起身。

3. 操作强度

（1）本节功法分左式和右式，两式操作次数必须保持一致，如左式操作3次，则右式也需操作3次，计算为本节功法操作了3次，以此类推。

（2）如果本节功法与全套功法一起操作，一般情况操作3次或6次。

如果单独操作本节功法，可以根据自身状况，按照3、6、9、12的次数递增运动量，直至身体微微汗出为度。

4. 功法作用

本节功法以左、右开弓的动作，分左式和右式操作，体现左右平衡之意，通过两式对等的操作次数和强度。一方面，训练身体左右两侧的软组织（肌肉、关节、韧带、筋膜、滑囊等），使两侧软组织的生物力协调一致，能够纠正机体左右失衡问题；另一方面，十二正经外行线呈左右对称分布，通过左右开弓对抗用力，可以调动、调和身体两侧的经络气血。

---

① 塌腰：躯体上身前屈状态，是造成腰部向后弓起的不正确体位。

2. Common Mistakes

(1) The foot and leg, when stepping forward, fail to be at a 45-degree angle toward the left or right front.

(2) The tiptoes fail to clutch inward on the ground after a step forward, causing the two feet imbalanced (toe out).

(3) Shrug shoulders and arch the back[1] when raising the arms; the two arms can't give an opposite force during drawing the bow, causing the chest to be forward and the hands to be feeble.

(4) In the movement of squatting and drawing the bow, the weight of the body fails to be shifted to the corresponding side (The body weight should be shifted to the left leg in the left posture and vice versa.), and meanwhile the upper body does not tilt slightly to the corresponding side (The upper body should tilt left in the left posture and vice versa.).

(5) During rising to your feet and putting the palms together, stand up directly before the body weight is shifted back to the midline of the body.

3. Amount of Qigong Exercises

(1) This routine is composed of the left and right postures. The practice amount of both sides should be consistent. For instance, if the left exercise is done 3 times, then the right one should be done 3 times. In this way it can be counted as practicing this routine for 3 times and so on.

(2) This routine, when performed together with a full set of Qigong exercises, is generally done 3 or 6 times.

When doing this routine alone, you can gradually increase the amount of exercise by 3, 6, 9 or 12 times according to your own condition until sweating slightly in your body.

4. Functions and Effects

This routine is practiced from side to side by acting as if drawing a bow left-handed and right-handed, which presents a balance between the left and the right by means of the equal amount of exercise on both sides. On the one hand, this routine helps to train the soft tissues (muscles, joints, ligaments, fascia, bursae, etc.) on the left and right sides of the body so as to make these soft tissues on both sides biomechanically coordinated and consistent, which can rectify the left-right imbalance of the body. On the other hand, the outer moving lines of the twelve regular meridians are symmetrically distributed. Drawing the bow left-handed and right-handed through the opposite strength can activate and regulate the qi and blood of the meridians on both sides of the body.

---

[1] arch the back (塌腰 tā yāo): a state of the upper body bent to the front, leading to an incorrect body posture with the waist arched backward

下蹲能够有效地增强下肢的肌肉力量，提高下肢的平衡和协调能力。两臂拉伸、转颈、上身倾斜，使颈、肩、上肢、腰部等部位的肌肉得到有效拉伸，可以缓解生理性疲劳，也有利于矫正驼背、肩内收等不良姿势，并能起到防治颈肩腰腿痛等软组织疾病的作用。

第三节　调理脾胃须单举

本节功法是在预备式的基础上，按照先左后右的顺序，左右两手交替托举进行操作的。

1. 调身操作步骤

（1）预备式（图1-3-1、图1-3-2）

两足跟并拢，脚尖外分。双手自然垂在身体两侧，目视远方，全身放松。

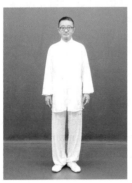 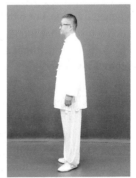

图1-3-1 (Fig.1-3-1)　　　图1-3-2 (Fig.1-3-2)

（2）左腕提起（图1-3-3）

左手腕关节微曲，掌心向后，指尖向下，沿体侧足少阳胆经，缓缓提起，至左侧髂棘高度，左肘关节内收。

右臂置于右侧，两肩关节下沉，全身放松。

Squatting can enhance the muscle strength of the lower limbs effectively and improve the balance and coordination of the lower limbs. Stretching the arms, turning the neck and tilting the upper body help to stretch the muscles of the neck, shoulders, upper limbs and waist effectively, which can alleviate physiological fatigue and correct bad postures such as hunchback and shoulder adduction as well. This practice is also conducive to the prevention and treatment of such soft tissue diseases as pains in the neck, shoulders, waist, legs and so on.

Routine 3   Holding One Arm Aloft Alternately to Regulate the Functions of the Spleen and Stomach

This routine is based on the preparatory posture and done with raising the left hand and the right hand alternately according to the sequence of left first and then right.

1. Step−by−step Instructions

(1) Preparatory posture (Fig.1-3-1, Fig.1-3-2)

Stand with heels together and tiptoes apart. Place both hands naturally alongside the body. Look straight ahead. Keep the whole body relaxed.

(2) Raising the left wrist (Fig.1-3-3)

Firstly, slightly bend the left wrist with the palm backward and fingers downward. Gradually raise the left wrist along the Gallbladder Meridian of Foot-*Shaoyang* to the level of the left iliac crest with the left elbow joint adducted.

Place the right arm on the right side of the body. Loosen up the shoulders and keep the whole body relaxed.

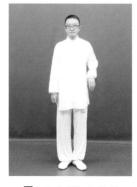

图1−3−3 (Fig.1−3−3)

（3）左掌上举（图1-3-4～图1-3-7）

左掌向外翻掌，使掌心向上，拇指指尖向外，四指指尖向前，手如托物，缓缓自体侧向体前上托，托至肩关节高度。

在肩关节水平，左掌以腕关节为轴，缓缓向前、前外、外、外后、内旋转，当旋转至外后时，左肘关节顺势外撑，继续旋腕，至拇指的指尖向前，四指的指尖向内（对准耳郭）。

与此同时，右侧肘关节外展，带动右侧腕关节内旋、背曲，使拇指向后，四指指尖向内，掌面与地面平行。

左手继续沿耳郭，缓缓上托，托至头顶，掌面与地面平行。左肘关节微曲（不可挺直），双目平视正前方。

保持此左托右按（即左掌在头顶部托举，右掌在体侧髂棘平面下按）的状态，停顿1个呼吸的时间（可默念1至5个数字，也可做1个腹式呼吸运动以度量时间）。

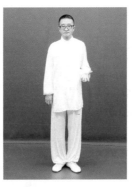 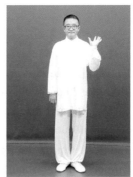

图1-3-4 (Fig.1-3-4)　　　图1-3-5 (Fig.1-3-5)

(3) Lifting the left palm (Fig.1-3-4 ~ Fig.1-3-7)

Rotate the left hand outward so that the palm faces upward. Keep the thumb outward and the other four fingertips forward. Push the palm skyward slowly along the side of the body toward the front of the body as if lifting an object to the shoulder level.

At the shoulder level, slowly rotate the left palm forward, outward, backward and inward with the wrist as an axis. When rotating the palm outward and backward, stretch the left elbow outward and continue to rotate the wrist until the tip of the thumb points forward with the other four fingertips inward (toward the auricle).

At the same time, stretch the right elbow outward, driving the right wrist to rotate inward and bend with the thumb backward, the other four fingertips inward and the palm parallel to the ground.

Continue to push the left palm upward along the auricle till up to the top of the head with the palm parallel to the ground. Keep the left elbow slightly bent (instead of erect). Look straight ahead.

Hold this position of left-handed lifting with right-handed pressing (i.e. lifting over the top of the head with the left hand while pressing down with the right hand alongside the iliac crest) and pause for one breath (counting silently from 1 to 5 or taking one abdominal breath to measure time).

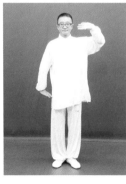 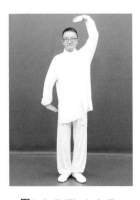

图1-3-6 (Fig.1-3-6)　　图1-3-7 (Fig.1-3-7)

（4）左落右托（图1-3-8、图1-3-9）

左臂缓缓沿体侧外展下落。同时，右臂放松，肘关节内收，腕关节回落至体侧。当左臂落至左侧肩关节高度时，右手腕关节微曲，掌心向后，指尖向下，沿体侧足少阳胆经平面，缓缓提起，提至右侧髂棘高度，右肘关节内收。

左臂继续沿体侧外展下落。同时，右掌向外翻掌，使掌心向上，拇指指尖向外，四指指尖向前，手如托物，缓缓自体侧向体前上托，托至右侧肩关节高度。此时，左臂缓缓落回体侧。

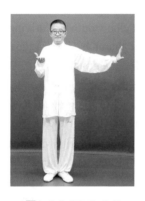 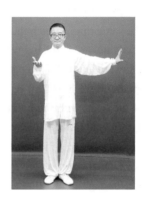

图1-3-8 (Fig.1-3-8)　　　　图1-3-9 (Fig.1-3-9)

（5）右掌上举（图1-3-10、图1-3-11）

右掌在肩关节水平，以腕关节为轴，缓缓向前、前外、外、外后、内进行旋转，当旋转至外后时，右肘关节顺势外撑，继续旋腕，至拇指指尖向前，四指指尖向内（对准耳郭）时，左肘关节外展，带动左腕关节内旋、背曲，使拇指向后，四指指尖向内，掌面与地面保持平行。

右手继续沿耳郭，缓缓上托，托至头顶，掌面与地面平行。右肘关节微曲（不可挺直），双目平视正前方。

保持此右托左按（即右掌在头顶部托举，左掌在体侧髂棘平面下按）的状态，停顿1个呼吸的时间（可默念1至5个数字，也可做1个腹式呼吸运动以度量时间）。

(4) Left arm falling with right-hand lifting (Fig.1-3-8, Fig.1-3-9)

Put down the left arm slowly alongside the body. Meanwhile, relax the right arm with the elbow adducted and the wrist back to the side of the body. As your left arm falls to the shoulder level, bend the right wrist slightly with the palm backward and the fingertips downward and raise it slowly along the Gallbladder Meridian of Foot-*Shaoyang* till up to the level of the iliac crest with the right elbow adducted.

The left arm proceeds to fall down along the side of the body. Meanwhile, rotate the right hand outward so that the palm faces upward. Keep the thumb outward and the fingers forward. Push the palm skyward slowly along the side of the body toward the front of the body as if lifting an object to the shoulder level. Simultaneously, the left arm goes slowly back to the side of the body.

(5) Lifting the right palm (Fig.1-3-10, Fig.1-3-11)

At the shoulder level, slowly rotate the right palm forward, outward, backward and inward with the wrist as an axis. When rotating the palm outward and backward, stretch the right elbow outward and continue to rotate the wrist until the thumb points forward with the other four fingertips inward (toward the auricle). Stretch the left elbow outward, driving the left wrist to rotate inward and bend with the thumb backward, the other four fingertips inward and the palm parallel to the ground.

Continue to push the right hand upward along the auricle till up to the top of the head with the palm parallel to the ground. Keep the right elbow slightly bent (instead of erect). Look straight ahead.

Hold this position of right-handed lifting with left-handed pressing (i.e. lifting over the top of the head with the right palm while pressing down with the left palm alongside the iliac crest) and pause for one breath (counting from 1 to 5 or taking one abdominal breath to measure time).

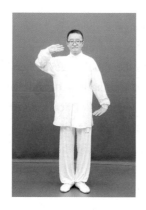 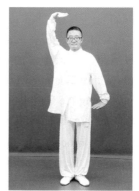

图1-3-10 (Fig.1-3-10)　　图1-3-11 (Fig.1-3-11)

（6）右落左托（图1-3-12）

右臂沿体侧外展下落。左掌外翻，掌心向上，上托至左侧肩关节高度。此时，右臂缓缓落回体侧。继续重复上述操作。

重复上述操作后，恢复到预备式。

2. 易犯错误

（1）单臂上举时耸肩、夹肩，造成手三阴、手三阳的经气阻滞不通。

（2）腕关节在耳郭部旋转时，不是用同侧肘关节的外展外旋带动腕关节旋转，而是腕关节主动旋转，容易造成腕关节的局部损伤。

（3）左托右按、右托左按时，两手对抗用力不对等，造成身体左右倾斜，不能保持中立位。

（4）单臂回落时，一方面肩关节、肘关节未能外展，不是在体侧回落而是在体前回落，另一方面回落速度过快，与另一侧托举配合不协调。

(6) Right arm falling with left-handed lifting (Fig.1-3-12)

Put down the right arm slowly alongside the body. Rotate the left hand outward with the palm up and raise it to the left shoulder level. Simultaneously, the right arm goes slowly back to the side of the body. Repeat this practice.

After the repetition of the above movements, return to the preparatory posture.

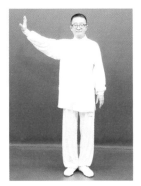

图1-3-12 (Fig.1-3-12)

2. Common Mistakes

(1) Shrugging and clamping the shoulders during holding one arm aloft may obstruct the free flow of qi of the three yin meridians of the hand and the three yang meridians of the hand.

(2) In the process of rotating the wrist alongside the auricle, the active rotation of the wrist instead of driving it to rotate with the ipsilateral elbow's extending force is liable to bring injuries to the wrist.

(3) In the movement of left-hand lifting with right-hand pressing or right-hand lifting with left-hand pressing, the opposite force applied by the two hands is not equal, causing the body to slant from side to side and not in a centered position.

(4) When putting down one arm, on the one hand, the failure in spreading the shoulder and the wrist outward causes the arm to fall in front of the body rather than alongside the body. On the other hand, the speed of putting down the arm is too fast to be in coordination with that of raising the arm on the other side.

（5）请在整个操作过程保持沉肩①、坠肘②的状态，一旦感觉肩背部酸痛不适时，及时纠正，做到不耸肩、不夹肩；腕关节旋转向上托举时，用同侧肘关节的外展外旋带动腕关节旋转上举，并保持与另一侧单臂的回落速度一致；左托右按、右托左按时，两手对抗用力要对等，以身体保持中立位、不向左或右倾斜为度；单臂回落时，要以肩关节、肘关节的外展动作，带动单臂沿体侧足少阳胆经回落。

3. 操作强度

（1）本节功法两臂托举、回落左右交替为1次操作。

（2）如果本节功法与全套功法一起操作，操作3次或6次。

（3）如果单独操作本节功法，可以根据自身状况，按照3、6、9、12的次数递增运动量，最多不超过12次。

4. 功法作用

本节功法冠名"调理脾胃"，是通过两臂的交替举、落和对抗牵拉，引动体内气机出现升降运动，而脾胃是体内气机升降的枢纽，因此，单臂交替升降运动引发的是中焦脾胃的清升浊降③功能。

另外，本节动作能够有效锻炼肩背部软组织的协调性，也可使脊柱各椎骨间的小关节及小肌肉得到锻炼，对脊柱的稳定性有帮助。

---

① 沉肩：肩关节放松，不被动耸起。
② 坠肘：肘关节放松，不向上架起。
③ 清升浊降：清升是营养物质升腾布散、营养全身；浊降是代谢的废物下降从二阴排出体外。

(5) Please relax the shoulders[1] and drop the elbows[2] all the time during the practice. Once you feel sore or uncomfortable on the shoulders and back, correct the wrong movements. Don't shrug or clamp the shoulders. As rotating the wrist and lifting it upward, remember to drive the wrist to rotate and lift with the external spread and rotation of the ipsilateral elbow and keep the same speed with the other arm's falling movement. In the movement of left-hand lifting with right -hand pressing or right-hand lifting with left-hand pressing, the opposite force applied by the two hands must be equal to keep the body in a centered position. Don't slant the body from side to side. When putting down one arm, bring it back to the Spleen Meridian of Foot-*Shaoyng* alongside the body with the external spreading force of the shoulder and the elbow.

3. Amount of Qigong Exercises

(1) In this routine, the alternative movements of lifting up and putting down the two arms are counted as doing the practice for one time.

(2) This routine, when performed together with a full set of Qigong exercises, is generally done 3 or 6 times.

(3) When doing this routine alone, you can gradually increase the amount of exercise by 3, 6, 9 or 12 times according to your own condition. Do it 12 times at most.

4. Functions and Effects

This routine, entitled "to regulate the functions of the spleen and stomach", is to induce the upward and downward movements of qi through lifting up and putting down the two arms alternatively and the opposite pulling strength. The spleen and stomach are considered as the pivot of the ascending and descending of qi movements in the body. Therefore, lifting up and putting down the two arms alternatively aims to enhance the function of ascending the lucid and descending the turbid[3] of the spleen and stomach in the middle energizer.

In addition, this routine can improve the coordination of the soft tissues of shoulders and back effectively, and also can exercise the small joints and small muscles between the vertebrae of the spine, which is helpful to maintain the stability of the spine.

---

① relax the shoulders (沉肩 chén jiān): keep the shoulders relaxed instead of hunched passively
② drop the elbows (坠肘 zhuì zhǒu): keep the elbow joints relaxed instead of raised up
③ ascending the lucid and descending the turbid: Ascending the lucid refers to the nutrient materials ascending and dispersing to nourish the whole body while descending the turbid refers to the metabolic wastes going down to be expelled out of the body through the urethral orifice and anus.

第四节　五劳七伤往后瞧

本节功法是在预备式的基础上，按照先左后右的顺序，左右两式交替进行操作。

1. 调身操作步骤

（1）预备式（图1-4-1、图1-4-2）

两足跟并拢，足尖外分。双手自然垂在身体两侧，目视远方，全身放松。

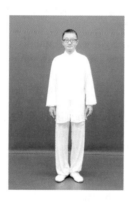 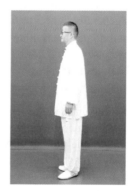

图1-4-1 (Fig.1-4-1)　　图1-4-2 (Fig.1-4-2)

（2）开步（图1-4-3）

重心移到左脚，右脚向右跨一步，两脚的宽度与两肩的宽度一致，两脚尖微微内扣，使两脚平行开立后，重心移回中线。

然后，身体保持中正，两脚站稳，五趾抓地，足跟踏实地面，膝关节挺直，保持双下肢不动，髋关节固定不移（之后上身旋转而髋关节仍不可移动）。

Routine 4   Looking Backward to Relieve Five Consumptions and Seven Impairments

This routine, based on the preparatory posture, starts with left first and then right. Both are practiced alternately in sequence.

1. Step–by–step Instructions

(1) Preparatory posture (Fig.1-4-1, Fig.1-4-2)

Stand with heels together and tiptoes apart. Place both hands alongside the body. Look straight ahead. Keep the whole body relaxed.

(2) Starting posture (Fig.1-4-3)

Shift the body weight to the left foot. Take a step right with the right foot, shoulder-width apart. Keep the tiptoes slightly clutched inward. After standing with the feet apart and parallel to each other, shift the body weight to the midline of the body.

Then, keep the body in a centered and upright position, stand firm, clutch the ground with the toes and hold the heels firm down on the ground. Keep the knees straight and upright, the legs and the hip joints unmovable (not moving the hip joints when turning the upper body).

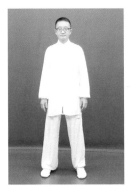

图1–4–3 (Fig.1–4–3)

（3）左式

右撑左贴（图1-4-4、图1-4-5）

右臂自体侧抬起，沉肩、坠肘、悬腕。

右手掌心向下，向前上方画弧，至膻中穴[1]高度，距离胸前30cm处，翻腕使掌心向前，虎口向下，肘关节屈曲外撑，使右臂围拢呈半圆。

左臂后撤，肘关节屈曲外展，掌心向后，虎口向上，将左掌背侧贴于第四腰椎处（腰阳关穴[2]）。

右臂前撑，以固定右侧躯体，左臂后贴，以固定左侧躯体，并稳定腰骶部，两臂争力，成向左转腰的趋势。

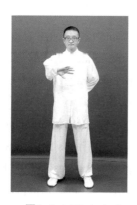 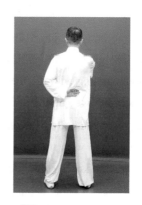

图1-4-4 (Fig.1-4-4)　　　图1-4-5 (Fig.1-4-5)

转腰侧屈（图1-4-6、图1-4-7）

接着，以第四、五腰椎为支点，以体中心线（百会穴[3]至会阴穴[4]一线）为轴，上身向左、左后缓缓水平磨转（如磨盘转动），磨转至最大限度（也就是如果再转动髋关节就会随之而动）。

然后，整个上身向左缓缓侧屈，保持头、颈、胸、腰整体不偏离中心线，侧屈至两眼的余光能够看到右侧的足跟为度。

---

① 膻中穴：属于任脉的穴位，位于体前正中线上，横平第4肋间隙，两乳头连线的中点。
② 腰阳关穴：属于督脉的穴位，位于后正中线上，第4腰椎棘突下凹陷中。
③ 百会穴：属于督脉的穴位，位于头顶正中心，两耳尖连线向上连线的中点处。
④ 会阴穴：属于任脉的穴位，位于前后二阴中间。

(3) The left posture

Pushing the right arm forward with the left arm against the back (Fig.1-4-4, Fig.1-4-5)

Raise the right arm along the side of the body with the shoulders relaxed, the elbow dropped and the wrist raised.

With the right palm downward, draw an arc forward till up to the level of Danzhong[1], 30 cm away from the chest, then turn the wrist to bring the palm forward and Hukou downward. Bend the elbow and extend it outward to hold the right arm in a semicircle.

Retract the left arm with the elbow bent and stretched outward, the palm backward and Hukou upward. Put the back of the left palm against the 4th lumbar vertebra (Yaoyangguan[2]).

Push the right arm forward to stabilize the right side of the body while putting the left arm against the back to stabilize the left side of the body. Keep the lumbosacral part stable. Exert an opposite force with the two arms to form a tendency of turning the waist left.

Turning the waist and bending sideways (Fig.1-4-6, Fig.1-4-7)

Then, with the 4th and 5th lumbar vertebrae as a supporting point and the midline of the body (from Baihui[3] to Huiyin[4]) as an axis, slowly turn the upper body left and backward horizontally (as if a millstone turns) to its maximum limitation (just before causing the hip joints to move).

Afterwards, bend the upper body to the left side slowly. Do not let the head, neck, chest and waist deviate from the center line. Bend laterally till the right heel can be seen from the corner of the eyes.

---

[1] Danzhong (CV17): an acupoint of the Conception Vessel, on the anterior midline of the body, on the level of the 4th intercostal space, at the midpoint of the line connecting both nipples

[2] Yaoyangguan (GV3): an acupoint of the Governor Vessel, on the posterior midline, in the depression below the spinous process of the 4th lumbar vertebra

[3] Baihui (GV20): an acupoint of the Governor Vessel, at the center of the head, at the midpoint of the line connecting the apices of both ears

[4] Huiyin (CV1): an acupoint of the Conception Vessel, on the perineum, at the midpoint between the posterior border of the scrotum and anus in male and between the posterior commissure of the large labia and anus in female

此时，停顿1个呼吸的时间（可默念1至5个数字，也可做1个腹式呼吸运动以度量时间）。

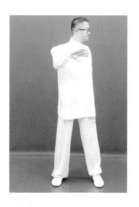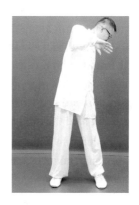

图1-4-6 (Fig.1-4-6)　　　　图1-4-7 (Fig.1-4-7)

起身回掌（图1-4-8）

上身缓缓向右侧屈，至整个身体恢复到中心线与地面垂直的位置。

然后，以第四、五腰椎为支点，以体中心线（百会穴至会阴穴一线）为轴，上身向右、右前缓缓水平磨转（如磨盘转动），磨转至面向正前方。

磨转的同时，双臂松力回撤至体侧，接右式。

（4）右式

左撑右贴（图1-4-9、图1-4-10）

左臂自体侧抬起，沉肩、坠肘、悬腕。

左手掌心向下，向前上方画弧，至膻中穴高度，距离胸前30cm处，翻腕使掌心向前，虎口向下，肘关节屈曲外撑，使左臂围拢呈半圆。

At this moment, pause for one breath (counting silently from 1 to 5 or taking one abdominal breath to measure time).

Turning the body back to the midline and adducting the palms (Fig.1-4-8)

Slowly bend the upper body right till the whole body gets back to the midline position, perpendicular to the ground.

Then, with the 4th and 5th lumbar vertebrae as a supporting point and the midline of the body (from Baihui to Huiyin) as an axis, slowly turn the upper body right and forward horizontally (as if a millstone turns) until facing straight ahead.

While swinging the body, loosen up both arms and get them back to the sides of the body, then continue from the right posture.

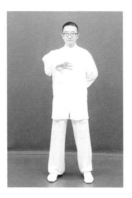

图1-4-8 (Fig.1-4-8)

(4) The right posture

Pushing the left arm forward with the right arm against the back (Fig.1-4-9, Fig.1-4-10)

Raise the left arm along the side of the body with the shoulders re-laxed, the elbow dropped and the wrist raised.

With the left palm down, draw an arc in the front till up to the level of Danzhong, 30 cm away from your chest, then turn the wrist to bring the palm forward and Hukou downward. Bend the elbow and extend it outward to hold the left arm in a semicircle.

右臂后撤，肘关节屈曲外展，掌心向后，虎口向上，将右掌背侧贴于第四腰椎处。

左臂前撑，右臂后贴，并稳定腰骶部，两臂争力，成向右转腰的趋势。

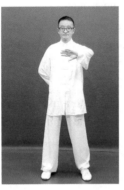
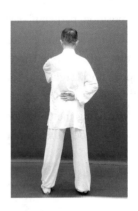

图1-4-9 (Fig.1-4-9)　　　　图1-4-10 (Fig.1-4-10)

转腰侧屈（图1-4-11、图1-4-12）

接着，以第四、五腰椎为支点，以体中心线为轴，上身向右、右后缓缓水平磨转，磨转至最大限度。

然后，整个上身向右缓缓侧屈，保持头、颈、胸、腰整体不偏离中心线，侧屈至两眼的余光能够看到左侧的足跟为度。

此时，停顿1个呼吸的时间。

起身回掌（图1-4-13）

上身缓缓向左侧屈，至整个身体恢复到中心线与地面垂直的位置。

然后，以第四、五腰椎为支点，以体中心线为轴，上身向左、左前缓缓水平磨转至面向正前方。

Retract the right arm with the elbow bent and stretched outward, the palm backward and Hukou upward. Put the back of the right palm against the 4th lumbar vertebra.

Push the left arm forward while putting the right arm against the back to keep the lumbosacral part stable. Exert an opposite force with the two arms to form a tendency of turning the waist right.

Turning the waist and bending sideways (Fig.1-4-11, Fig.1-4-12)

Then, with the 4th and 5th lumbar vertebrae as a supporting point and the midline of the body as an axis, slowly turn the upper body right and backward horizontally to its maximum limitation.

Afterwards, bend the upper body to the right side slowly. Do not let the head, neck, chest and waist deviate from the center line. Bend laterally till the left heel can be seen from the corner of the eyes.

At this moment, pause for one breath.

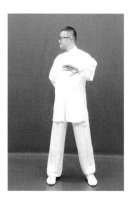
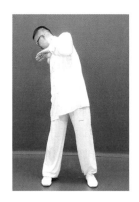

图1-4-11(Fig.1-4-11)   图1-4-12 (Fig.1-4-12)

Turning the body back to the midline and adducting the palms (Fig.1-4-13)

Slowly bend the upper body left till the whole body gets back to the midline position, perpendicular to the ground.

Then, with the 4th and 5th lumbar vertebrae as a supporting point and the midline of the body as an axis, slowly turn the upper body left and forward horizontally until facing straight ahead.

磨转的同时，双臂松力回撤至体侧。恢复到预备式。

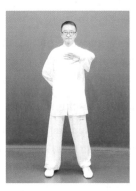

图1-4-13 (Fig.1-4-13)

2. 易犯错误

（1）操作右撑左贴或左撑右贴时，不能把握撑和贴的操作内涵，仅是将双臂一前一后置于身体的前后位置，未能将双臂的肩关节、肘关节、腕关节充分外展，两臂肘关节不能形成前后对抗之势，达不到稳定躯干和脊柱的目的。

（2）转腰侧屈的过程中，一是随腰骶部的旋转，两侧髋关节出现左右旋转、屈髋等动作，两侧膝关节屈曲，两腿不能挺直，双足不能踏实地面；二是上身侧屈变成了弯腰驼背，达不到牵拉脊柱两侧的竖脊肌及第四、五腰椎附近软组织的目的。

（3）起身回掌过程中，上身没有恢复到中立位，就急着向正前方磨转，或转体、起身过快，容易造成腰骶部软组织的扭挫伤。

3. 操作强度

本节功法左右交替磨转为1次操作。

如果本节功法与全套功法一起操作，一般情况左右交替，各操作3次或6次。

如果单独操作本节功法，可以根据自身状况，左右交替，按照3、6、9、12的次数递增运动量，最多不超过12次。

048

While swinging the body, loosen up both arms and get them back to the side of the body. Return to the preparatory posture.

2. Common Mistakes

(1) Fail to grasp the key to the practice of pushing the right arm forward with the left arm against the back or pushing the left arm forward with the right arm against the back. Just only place one arm in the front and the other in the back rather than fully stretch the shoulders, elbows and wrists outward. As a result, the two elbows are unable to exert opposite forces so that the purpose of keeping the body and the spine firm is not achieved.

(2) During turning the waist and bending sideways, firstly, the hip joints are turned and bent from side to side with the rotation of the lumbosacral part. The knees and legs are not straightened and the feet are not firm on the ground. Secondly, bending the body sideways is liable to hunch over so as to fail to attain the aim of fully pulling the erector spinae and the soft tissues near the 4th and 5th lumbar vertebrae.

(3) In the process of turning the body back to the midline and adducting the palms, turning to the front in a hurry before coming back to the midline, or turning around and rising to your feet too fast may cause injuries to the lumbosacral soft issues.

3. Amount of Qigong Exercises

In this routine, the alternative movements of turning the body to the left and then to the right are counted as doing the practice for one time.

This routine, when performed together with a full set of Qigong exercises, is generally done 3 or 6 times.

When doing this routine alone, you can gradually increase the amount of exercise by 3, 6, 9 or 12 times according to your own condition. Do it 12 times at most.

4.功法作用

本节功法冠名"五劳七伤"，有五劳和七伤两层含义。

关于五劳，《素问·宣明五气》曰："久视伤血，久卧伤气，久坐伤肉，久立伤骨，久行伤筋，是谓五劳所伤。"指出日常的行为过度，会造成气、血、肉、骨、筋的损伤。《诸病源候论·虚劳病诸候》提出了虚劳五候，即肺劳、肝劳、心劳、脾劳、肾劳，是从五脏虚劳的角度认识五劳的。两者提出的五劳，字面上有区别，然而从肺主气、心主血脉、脾主肌肉、肝主筋、肾主骨的角度看，虽然两者的表达方式不同，但核心内容是一致的。可以理解为，五劳的外伤在气、血、肉、骨、筋，内伤在肺、心、脾、肾、肝。

关于七伤，《金匮要略·血痹虚劳病脉证并治》曰："食伤、忧伤、饮伤、房室伤、饥伤、劳伤、经络营卫气伤，合为七伤。"另外生活当中有"大饱伤脾，大怒气逆伤肝，强力举重久坐湿地伤肾，形寒饮冷伤肺，形劳意损伤神，风雨寒暑伤形，恐惧不节伤志"的说法。两种表述（内外）特点基本一致，而七伤更偏重于与日常生活的习惯与规律关系密切。

4. Functions and Effects

This routine, entitled "Five Consumptions and Seven Impairments", contains Wu Lao (Five Consumptions) and Qi Shang (Seven Impairments).

As for the five consumptions, in *Plain Questions· Discussion on the Elucidation of Five-Qi* (Sù Wèn·Xuān Míng Wǔ Qì, 素问·宣明五气), it says, " Seeing for a long time impairs the blood; sleeping for a long time impairs the qi; sitting for a long time impairs the muscles; standing for a long time impairs the bones; and walking for a long time impairs the sinews. These are the damages caused by five kinds of overstrain." It points out that excessive daily activities may cause injuries to qi, blood, fleshes, bones and sinews. *Treatise on Causes and Manifestations of Diseases· Consumptive Diseases* (Zhū Bìng Yuán Hòu Lùn · Xū Láo Bìng Zhū Hòu, 诸病源候论 · 虚劳病诸候) puts forward the five kinds of consumptive diseases including lung consumption, liver consumption, heart consumption, spleen consumption and kidney consumption, which are known from the perspective of the five-*zang* consumptions. The five consumptions mentioned in the two books are literally different. They are different in expression but essentially the same in the core concept from the perspective of the lung governing qi, the heart governing the blood and blood vessels, the spleen governing the fleshes, the liver governing the sinews and the kidney governing the bones. It can be understood that externally, the five consumptions do harm to qi, blood, fleshes, bones and sinews, but internally, they impair the lungs, heart, spleen, kidneys and liver.

As for the seven impairments, *Essentials of the Golden Cabinet· Blood Impediment and Consumptive Disease: Pulses, Patterns and Treatment* (Jīn Guì Yào Lüè· Xuè Bì Xū Láo Bìng Mài Zhèng Bìng Zhì, 金匮要略 · 血痹虚劳病脉证并治) states, "Damages caused by food, anxiety, drinking, sexual intercourse, hunger, overexertion and the damage of meridians, collaterals, nutrient qi and defensive qi are called seven impairments." In addition, as the saying goes, "Overeating impairs the spleen. Rage causes the reverse flow of qi and impairs the liver. Excessive weightlifting and sitting at the humid place for an extended period impair the kidneys. A cold body and chilled beverages impair the lungs. Physical overstrain and mental fatigue impair the spirit. The abnormal change of wind, rain, cold and heat impairs the body. Fear and excessive sexual activities impair the will (kidney)." The characteristics of the two statements (internal and external) are basically the same, while the seven impairments are more closely related to the habits and rules of daily life.

劳，有"痨"之说，以久之为病机，体现在"虚"。伤，虽有损伤积累的意思，但着重表现为突发、迅猛的特点，病机为急发，体现在"实"。可见，五劳与七伤合起来，泛指各种虚实病证。

为什么要"往后瞧"呢？也就是说，五劳七伤的康复要点"往后瞧"是关键。这是因为第四、五腰椎平面居于人体直立位横切面的正中间，是各种损伤的结点区域，而此平面以下的空间是任脉①、督脉②、冲脉③三条奇经共同的起点区域（一源三歧），也是五脏六腑积劳后气血瘀阻、病邪聚结的关键部位。

因此，"往后瞧"的操作，可将整个脊柱，以腰骶部为支点，进行充分全面的旋转、拉伸，在带动两侧的骨骼和软组织协调运动的基础上，加强深层韧带、小关节的运动，加强深层组织的气血供给，以改善久劳积伤之疾。同时，胸腹部与背腰部的协同磨转运动，能够有效刺激胸腹部的募穴④和腰背部的背俞穴⑤、夹脊穴⑥等，从而对五脏六腑的功能起到调节作用，达到内外同调的目的。

---

① 任脉：起于小腹内，下出于会阴部，向前上行于阴毛部，循腹沿体前正中线上行，至咽喉，再上行环绕口唇，经面部进入目眶下，联系于目。
② 督脉：起于小腹内，下行于会阴部，向后从尾骨端上行于脊柱的内部，上达项后风府，进入脑内，上行至头部颠顶，沿前额下行鼻柱，止于上唇系带处。
③ 冲脉：起于小腹内，下出于会阴部，向上行于脊柱内，其外行部分，经股动脉波动处与足少阴经交会，沿腹部两侧上行，至胸中散开，继而上达咽喉，环绕口唇。
④ 募穴：募，是聚集、汇合之意，募穴是脏腑之气汇聚于胸腹部的穴位。
⑤ 背俞穴：俞，是输注、转输之意，俞穴是脏腑之气输注于背腰部的穴位。
⑥ 夹脊穴：属于经外奇穴，位于背腰部脊柱两侧，第1胸椎至第5腰椎棘突下，后正中线旁开0.5寸，每侧17个穴位。

Consumption (láo, 劳), associated with "consumptive disease"(láo, 痨), takes the chronic as its pathogenesis and is manifested as "deficiency". Impairment, with the meaning of injury accumulation, is mainly characterized by a sudden and rapid onset. It takes the acute as its pathogenesis and is manifested as "excess". It can be seen that the five consumptions and seven impairments generally refer to all kinds of deficiency and excess syndromes.

Why do we need to "look backward"? In other words, the key to a recovery from the five consumptions and seven impairments is to "look backward". This is because the fourth and fifth lumbar vertebrae are located just at the center of the transection in the basic standing posture, which is considered as the node area of various injuries. The space below this transection is the common starting point of the Conception Vessel[1], the Governor Vessel[2] and the Thoroughfare Vessel[3] (known as "three vessels with one shared source"). It is also a key position where qi-blood stasis and obstruction occur and pathogens gather as a result of the overworked five *zang*-organs and six *fu*-organs.

Therefore, the "looking backward" movement can fully rotate and stretch the whole spine with the lumbar vertebrae as a supporting point, driving the coordinated movements of bones and soft tissues on both sides. It helps to enhance the movements of deep ligaments and facet joints and strengthen the supply of qi and blood for the deep tissues, finally to improve the symptoms caused by the injuries due to chronic overexertion. Meanwhile, the movement of turning the chest, abdomen, back and waist horizontally can effectively stimulate the Alarm Point[4] on the chest and abdomen and the Back Transport Points[5] and Jiaji[6] on the back, which will further regulate the functions of the five *zang*-organs and the six *fu*-organs.

---

[1] Conception Vessel: Conception Vessel (CV) starts from the lower abdomen, goes down to the perineum and runs upward to the pubes along the abdomen of the anterior midline and onto the throat. Then it moves upward, encircles the mouth and, along the face, enters the eyes.
[2] Governor Vessel: Governor Vessel (GV) starts from the lower abdomen, moves downward to the perineum, runs upward from the coccyx to the interior of the spine, reaches Fengfu (GV16) on the nape and enters the brain. Then it moves up to the top of the head, goes down along the forehead to the nose bridge and terminates at the upper labial frenum.
[3] Thoroughfare Vessel: Thoroughfare Vessel (TV) starts from the lower abdomen, goes down to the perineum and runs upward to the interior of the spine. Moving externally, it intersects the Meridian of Food-*Shaoyin* through the femoral artery, runs upward along both sides of the abdomen to the chest and disperse. Then it reaches the throat and encircles the mouth.
[4] Alarm Point (募穴 mù xué): The word 募 (mù) in Chinese has the meaning of "gathering or converging". Here it refers to the acupoint where the qi of the *zang-fu* organs converges in the chest and abdomen.
[5] Back Transport Points (背俞穴 bèi shù xué): The word 俞 (shù) in Chinese has the meaning of "transmitting". Here it refers to the acupoint where the qi of the *zang-fu* organs is transmitted into the back and waist.
[6] Jiaji (EX-B2): one of the extra acupoints, on both sides of the spine at the back and waist, below the spinous processes from the 1st thoracic vertebra to the 5th lumbar vertebra, 0.5 cun lateral to the posterior midline, with 17 acupoints on each side

第五节　摇头摆尾去心火

本节功法分左式和右式两式，是在预备式的基础上，按照先左后右的顺序，左右两式交替进行操作。

1. 调身操作步骤

（1）预备式（图1-5-1、图1-5-2）

两足跟并拢，脚尖外分。双手自然垂在身体两侧，目视远方，全身放松。

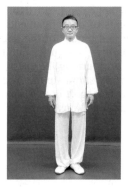 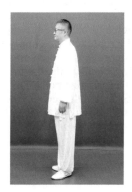

图1-5-1 (Fig.1-5-1)　　　　图1-5-2 (Fig.1-5-2)

（2）开步（图1-5-3）

重心移到右脚，向左跨开一大步，两脚的宽度是两肩宽度的1.5倍，两脚尖微微内扣，使两脚平行开立后，重心移至体正中线，膝关节微曲。

Routine 5   Swinging the Head and Lowering the Body to Eliminate Stress-induced Heart Fire

This routine includes the left and right postures. It is based on the preparatory posture and starts with left first and then right. Both are practiced alternately in sequence.

1. Step-by-step Instructions

(1) Preparatory posture (Fig.1-5-1, Fig.1-5-2)

Stand with heels together and tiptoes apart. Place both hands alongside the body. Look straight ahead. Keep the whole body relaxed.

(2) Starting posture (Fig.1-5-3)

Shift the body weight to the right foot. Take a big step to the left 1.5 times as wide as the shoulders. Keep the tiptoes slightly clutched inward. After standing with the feet apart and parallel to each other, shift the body weight to the midline of the body with the knees slightly bent.

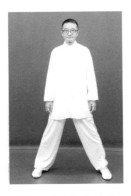

图1-5-3 (Fig.1-5-3)

（3）左式

俯身左转（图1-5-4～图1-5-6）

两臂沿体前抬起，沉肩、坠肘、悬腕。腕关节抬至肩关节高度时，上身前俯，同时，两臂缓缓下落，当俯身至背腰部与地面平行时，两臂自然垂于体前。

上身在俯身的平面，向左缓缓旋转90°。同时，左脚以脚跟为轴，脚尖随之向左侧转动90°。

左腿屈膝成直角，右腿微微蹬直，重心从两腿之间移至左腿上，成前弓后蹬之势。

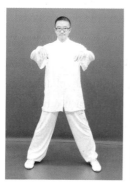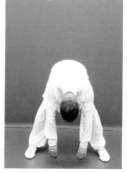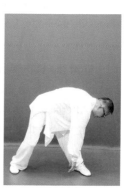

图1-5-4 (Fig.1-5-4)　　　图1-5-5 (Fig.1-5-5)　　　图1-5-6 (Fig.1-5-6)

右撑左按（图1-5-7、图1-5-8）

右臂向前抬起，至胸前膻中穴高度，右掌外旋，掌心向前，顺势向前推出，肘关节外展外旋，至手臂围拢呈半圆；同时，左侧肘关节微抬，腕关节背曲，使掌心向下、指尖向前，呈下按式，置于左侧大腿旁（距离左腿约一拳距离）。

两臂的肘关节对抗争力，头、颈、背、腰协同用力，上身缓缓起身，使之与右腿在同一斜平面上（与地面呈45°角）。目视前方，动作稍停，稳定重心。

(3) The left posture

Stooping down and turning left (Fig.1-5-4~Fig.1-5-6)

Raise the arms in front of the body with shoulders relaxed, elbows dropped and wrists raised. When lifting the wrists to the shoulder level, bend the upper body forward with both hands slowly down. Stoop down till the back and the waist are parallel to the ground, then let both arms hang down naturally in front of the body.

At the stooping level, slowly turn the upper body left to 90°. At the same time, turn the tiptoes left to 90° with the left heel as an axis.

Bend the left knee to 90°. Slightly straighten the right leg. Shift the body weight to the left leg in a front-bowing and back-pushing form.

Right arm pushing and left-handed pressing (Fig.1-5-7, Fig.1-5-8)

Raise the right arm forward to Danzhong. Rotate the right palm outward with the palm forward and push it ahead. Stretch and turn the elbow outward till your arm is held in a semicircle. At the same time, raise the left elbow slightly with the wrist bent, the palm down and the fingertips forward in a downward pressing form, and place it by the left thigh (one fist-width away from the left thigh).

The two elbows exert an opposite strength with the cooperation of the head, neck, back and waist. Raise the upper body slowly, keeping it parallel to the right leg (at a 45-degree angle to the ground). Look straight ahead. Hold this position for a moment and keep the body weight stabilized.

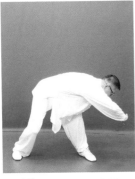
图1-5-7 (Fig.1-5-7)

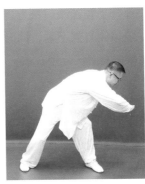
图1-5-8 (Fig.1-5-8)

摇头摆尾（图1-5-9）

以腰骶部为轴，下颌微微内收，头部缓缓向左上方旋转。利用头部旋转的力量，带动胸椎、腰椎、骶椎和尾椎向左缓缓旋转。

当感觉到尾椎部位受到旋转牵拉时，目视后上方，停顿1个呼吸的时间（可默念1至5个数字，或做1个腹式呼吸运动以度量时间）。

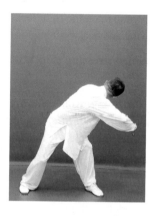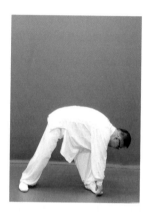

图1-5-9 (Fig.1-5-9)　　图1-5-10 (Fig.1-5-10)

松力回旋（图1-5-10）

头部带动颈部缓缓松力，恢复到右撑左按的状态。两臂缓缓回撤，至体侧自然下垂，同时，上身前俯，至背腰部与地面平行时，缓缓向右磨转，接右式。

（4）右式

俯身右转（图1-5-11～图1-5-12）

上身在俯身的平面，向右缓缓旋转180°。同时，右脚以脚跟为轴，脚尖随之向右侧转动。右腿屈膝成直角，左腿微微蹬直，重心从两腿之间移到右腿上，呈前弓后蹬之势。

Swinging the head and lowering the body (Fig.1-5-9)

Taking the lumbosacral part as an axis, slowly turn the head to the top left with the chin slightly adducted. Turn the thoracic vertebrae, the lumbar vertebrae, the sacral vertebrae and the caudal vertebrae to the left with the assistance of the head rotation.

When feeling a pull at the caudal vertebrae, look backward and upward and pause for one breath (counting silently from 1 to 5 or taking one abdominal breath to measure time).

Loosening and adducting (Fig.1-5-10)

Bring the neck into a loose state gradually with the help of the head and revert to the form of right arm pushing and left-handed pressing. Adduct the arms slowly, hanging them down naturally alongside the body. Meanwhile, bend the upper body forward till the back and the waist are parallel to the ground, then swing it to the right slowly. Then continue from the right posture.

(4) The right posture

Stooping down and turning right (Fig.1-5-11, Fig.1-5-12)

At the stooping level, slowly turn the upper body right to 180°. At the same time, turn the tiptoes right with the right heel as an axis. Bend the right knee to 90°. Slightly straighten the left leg. Shift the body weight to the right leg in a front-bowing and back-pushing form.

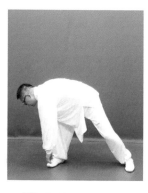
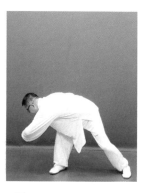

图1-5-11 (Fig.1-5-11)   图1-5-12 (Fig.1-5-12)

左撑右按（图1–5–13）

左臂向前抬起，至胸前膻中穴高度，左掌外旋，掌心向前，顺势向前推出，肘关节外展外旋，至手臂围拢呈半圆时，右侧肘关节微抬，腕关节背曲，使掌心向下、指尖向前，呈下按式，置于右侧大腿旁（距离右腿约一拳距离）。

两臂的肘关节对抗争力，头、颈、背、腰协同用力，上身缓缓起身，使之与左腿在同一斜平面上（与地面呈45°角）。目视前方，动作稍停，稳定重心。

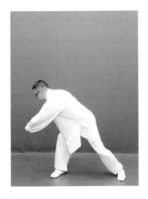 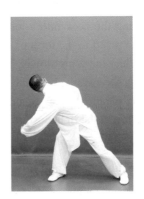

图1–5–13 (Fig.1–5–13)　　　　图1–5–14 (Fig.1–5–14)

摇头摆尾（图1–5–14）

以腰骶部为轴，下颌微微内收，头部缓缓向右上方旋转。利用头部旋转的力量，带动胸椎、腰椎、骶椎和尾椎向右缓缓旋转。

当感觉到尾椎部位受到旋转牵拉时，目视后上方，停顿1个呼吸的时间（可默念1至5个数字，或做1个腹式呼吸运动以度量时间）。

松力回旋（图1–5–15）

头部带动颈部缓缓松力，恢复到左撑右按的状态。两臂缓缓回撤，至体侧自然下垂，同时，上身前俯，至背腰部与地面平行时，缓缓向左磨转。

Left arm pushing and right-handed pressing (Fig.1-5-13)

Raise the left arm forward to Danzhong. Rotate the left palm outward with the palm forward and push it ahead. Stretch and turn the elbow outward till the arm is held in a semicircle. At the same time, raise the right elbow slightly with the wrist bent, the palm down and the fingertips forward in a downward pressing form, and place it by the right thigh (one fist-width away from the right thigh).

The two elbows exert an opposite strength with the cooperation of the head, neck, back and waist. Raise the upper body slowly, keeping it parallel to the left leg (at a 45-degree angle to the ground). Look straight ahead. Hold this position for a moment and keep the body weight stabilized.

Swinging the head and lowering the body (Fig.1-5-14)

Taking the lumbosacral part as an axis, turn the head slowly to the top right with the chin slightly adducted. Turn the thoracic vertebrae, the lumbar vertebrae, the sacral vertebrae and the caudal vertebrae to the right with the assistance of the head rotation.

When feeling a pull at the caudal vertebrae, look backward and upward and pause for one breath (counting silently from 1 to 5 or taking one abdominal breath to measure time).

Loosening and adducting (Fig.1-5-15)

Bring the neck into a loose state gradually with the help of the head and revert to the form of left arm pushing and right-handed pressing. Adduct the arms slowly, hanging them down naturally alongside the body. Meanwhile, bend the upper body forward till the back and the waist are parallel to the ground, then swing it to the left slowly.

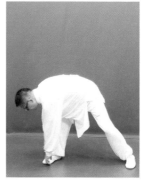

图1-5-15(Fig.1-5-15)

（5）收式（图1-5-16～图1-5-22）

松力回撤至正前方。

上身起身，同时，两臂沿体侧向外缓缓画圆展出，双手中指于头顶部相接，重心移到右腿，左腿收回一大步，足跟并拢。

两手掌心向下，沿体前中线缓缓下落至身体两侧。

恢复到预备式。

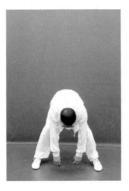
图1-5-16 (Fig.1-5-16)

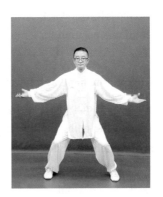
图1-5-17 (Fig.1-5-17)

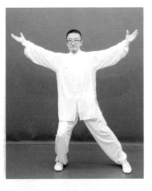
图1-5-18 (Fig.1-5-18)

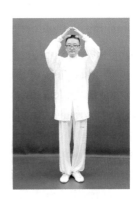
图1-5-19 (Fig.1-5-19)

(5) Closing form (Fig.1-5-16～Fig.1-5-22)

Loosen up and turn back to the straight front.

Raise the upper body. Alongside the body, stretch the arms outward slowly like drawing a circle. The two middle fingers of the hands meet at the top of the head. Shift the body weight to the right leg while retracting the left leg. Then bring the heels together.

With palms downward, put down the hands slowly to the sides of the body along the midline in front of the body.

Return to the preparatory posture.

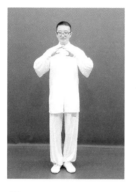

图1–5–20 (Fig.1–5–20)

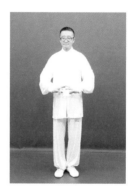

图1–5–21 (Fig.1–5–21)

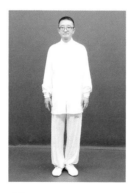

图1–5–22 (Fig.1–5–22)

2. 易犯错误

（1）俯身左转或俯身右转，两膝关节过于僵直紧张，足尖不能随上身的左右磨转而转换方向。

（2）右撑左按或左撑右按，两腕关节未能背曲、两肘关节外展外撑的对抗力不足，致使两臂不能稳定上身，不能以腰为轴保持上身进一步磨转。

（3）松力回旋，向左或向右转动时，足尖未能收回，就向另一方向磨转，造成整体动作不协调。

3. 操作强度

本节功法左右交替为1次操作。

如果本节功法与全套功法一起操作，一般情况左右交替，各操作3次或6次。

如果单独操作本节功法，可以根据自身状况，左右交替，按照3、6、9、12的次数递增运动量，最多不超过12次。

4. 功法作用

本节功法冠名"摇头摆尾"，是通过躯体的协调运动，运用头部顶旋动作，自上而下带动颈椎、胸椎、腰椎、骶尾椎进行旋转，最大限度地左右旋转整个脊柱，一方面直接将力量应用到脊柱侧弯、前后失衡的调整上，对脊柱病有很好的康复作用；另一方面牵拉脊柱周围的软组织，对脊柱的供血机制起到良好的促进作用，以加强脊柱及脊柱周围组织的气血运行，改善局部软组织的缺血缺氧，对脊柱两侧的软组织恢复生物力学平衡非常重要。

2. Common Mistakes

(1) In the movement of stooping down and turning left or right, the knees are so stiff and tense that the tiptoes fail to change the direction with the left and right swinging movements of the upper body.

(2) In the process of right arm pushing and left-handed pressing or left arm pushing and right-handed pressing, the wrists are not bent and the opposite strength exerted by stretching the elbows outward is not so strong that the arms can't stabilize the upper body. Moreover, the upper body fails to make a further swinging movement with the waist as an axis.

(3) During the loosening and adducting movements, when turning the body left or right, swinging to the other side without adducting the tiptoes makes the whole movement uncoordinated.

3. Amount of Qigong Exercises

Doing this routine alternatively from side to side is counted as practicing it for one time.

This routine, when performed together with a full set of Qigong exercises, is generally done 3 or 6 times.

When doing this routine alone, you can gradually increase the amount of exercise by 3, 6, 9 or 12 times according to your own condition. Do it 12 times at most.

4. Functions and Effects

This routine, entitled "swinging the head and lowering the body", is to rotate the cervical vertebrae, the thoracic vertebrae, the lumbar vertebrae and the caudal vertebrae from top to bottom through the coordinated movements of the body and the swing of the head. It can rotate the whole spine left and right to its maximum limitation. On the one hand, this routine applies the strength directly to the adjustment of the scoliosis and the anterior-posterior imbalance, which can promote the recovery of spinal diseases. On the other hand, by pulling the soft tissues around the spine, this routine promotes the blood supply, enhances the circulation of qi and blood around the spine and improves the ischemia and hypoxia of some soft tissues. Therefore, it plays an important role in restoring the biomechanical balance of the soft tissues around the spine.

脊柱与督脉、足太阳膀胱经的关系极为密切，而这两条经脉都与脑有直接的联系，"督脉，入络于脑"，"足太阳膀胱经，从颠入络脑"，所以本节功法对脊柱及脊柱周围组织的牵引拉伸作用本身直接影响了两条经脉的气血运行，进而对心脑的供血有很好的促进作用，其冠名"去心火"的真实意义就在于此。脑为元神之府，气血上荣于脑，神明得安，心火自然得除。久练此节功法，能够起到安神解郁，聪脑明目的作用。

第六节　两手攀足固肾腰

1. 调身操作步骤

（1）预备式（图1-6-1、图1-6-2）

足跟并拢，脚尖外分。双手自然垂在身体两侧，目视远方，全身放松。

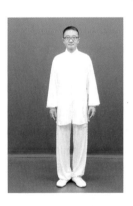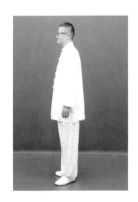

图1-6-1 (Fig.1-6-1)　　　图1-6-2 (Fig.1-6-2)

（2）展翅扩胸（图1-6-3～图1-6-5）

两手自体侧向前外侧展开，用肩关节的力量带动前臂在胸前向上、向外、向后展出。

同时，胸部向外、向上扩展，沉肩、坠肘、悬腕。

The spine is closely related to the Governor Vessel and the Bladder
Meridian of Foot-*Taiyang*. These two meridians are directly associated
with the brain. As described in TCM, "The Governor Vessel enters the
brain", "The Bladder Meridian of Foot-*Taiyang* enters the brain from
the top of the head." So, the traction effect in this routine on the spine
and the tissues around it directly influences the qi and blood circulation
of the two meridians, and thus can promote the blood supply to the heart
and brain. That's the true meaning of "Qu Xin Huo" (eliminating heart
fire). The brain is the palace of the original spirit. Qi and blood can
nourish the brain and make the spirit and mind relaxed and tranquilized.
As a result, the stress-induced heart fire will be eliminated gradually. A
persistent practice of this routine helps to tranquilize the mind, remove
stagnation, train the brain and improve the eyesight.

Routine 6   Moving the Hands Down and Touching the Feet to Strengthen the Kidney and Waist

1.Step–by–step Instructions

(1) Preparatory posture (Fig.1-6-1-, Fig.1-6-2)

Stand with heels together and tiptoes apart. Place both hands
alongside the body. Look straight ahead. Keep the whole body relaxed.

(2) Spreading the arms and expanding the chest (Fig.1-6-3～Fig.1-6-5)

Stretch both hands forward and outward from the sides of the
body. Through the strength of shoulders, drive the forearms to spread
upward, outward and backward in front of the chest.

Meanwhile, expand the chest outward and upward with shoulders
relaxed, elbows dropped and wrists raised.

当双臂提至肩关节高度时，双掌向外旋转，使掌心向上，大指向后，四指向外。

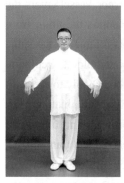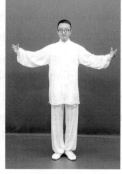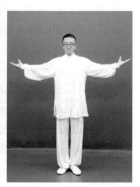

图1-6-3（Fig.1-6-3）　　　　图1-6-4（Fig.1-6-4）　　　　图1-6-5（Fig.1-6-5）

（3）俯身下按（图1-6-6～图1-6-10）

两手缓缓内收，至体前正中线将两中指中冲穴相接（与印堂穴①等高），两掌微微内合。双手合十后，沿体前正中线（任脉），缓缓下落。

当落至膻中穴的高度时，上身缓缓前俯，俯身至上身与地面平行，同时双腿要并拢、挺直。

上身继续向下俯身，尽量向双腿靠近，同时双手继续下按。

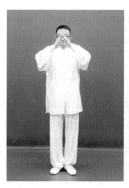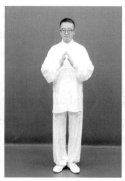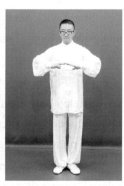

图1-6-6 (Fig.1-6-6)　　　　图1-6-7 (Fig.1-6-7)　　　　图1-6-8 (Fig.1-6-8)

①印堂穴：属于经外奇穴，位于人体额部，在两眉头的中间。

When the arms are raised to the shoulder level, rotate both hands outward with the palms upward, the thumbs backward and the rest fingers outward.

(3) Stooping down and pressing the hands downward (Fig.1-6-6~Fig.1-6-10)

Adduct both hands slowly to the midline in front of the body and then connect the middle fingers at Zhongchong (level with Yintang[1]) with the palms slightly joined. With the hands put together, bring them down slowly along the midline (Conception Vessel) in front of the body.

With the hands down to Danzhong, slowly bend the upper body forward and stoop down till it is parallel to the ground. Meanwhile, keep both legs together and straight.

Continue to stoop down the upper body further as close to the legs as possible. Meanwhile, keep the hands in a downward pressing position.

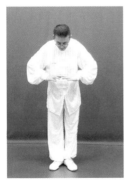
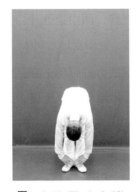

图1-6-9 (Fig.1-6-9)   图1-6-10 (Fig.1-6-10)

---

[1] Yintang (EX-HN3): one of the extra acupoints, on the forehead, at the midpoint between the eyebrows

（4）攀足挺臀（图1-6-11）

双掌向外平伸，中指相接，缓缓下按至双足，尽量使掌面接触足背侧。同时，臀部向后上方挺起，牵拉双腿足太阳膀胱经（此时两足踏实地面，不可抬起）。

当感觉到足跟部受到牵拉后，停顿1个呼吸的时间（可默念1至5个数字，也可做1个腹式呼吸运动以度量时间）。

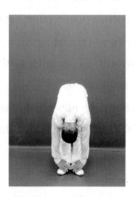

图1-6-11 (Fig.1-6-11)

（5）垂掌竖腰（图1-6-12～图1-6-14）

双手沉腕，两中指分开，十指自然下垂，两掌背相对，保持一拳的距离，置于双足之间。

用腰部的力量带动上身，缓缓向上起身，双臂随身体起来的同时，缓缓沿双腿中间上提。当上身恢复到直立位时，双手置于身体两侧。

(4) Hands touching the feet with the buttocks up (Fig.1-6-11)

Stretch both palms outward horizontally with the two middle fingers connected. Then press the palms slowly down to the feet as close to the dorsa of the feet as possible. Meanwhile, raise up the buttocks to pull Bladder Meridians of Foot–*Taiyang* of both legs (two feet firm on the ground and not off the ground).

When feeling a pull at the heels, pause for one breath (counting silently from 1 to 5 or taking one abdominal breath to measure time).

(5) Palms hanging down with the waist upright (Fig.1-6-12~Fig.1-6-14)

Keep the wrists down with the two middle fingers apart. Hang the ten fingers naturally with the hand backs facing each other, one fist-width away from each other and then place them between the feet.

Through the strength of the waist, raise the upper body slowly. Along with the upper body raised, slowly lift the arms along the midline of the legs.

When the upper body returns to the upright position, place your hands alongside the body.

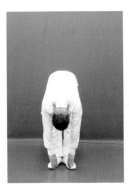 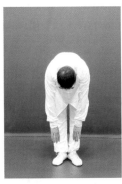 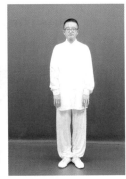

图1–6–12 (Fig.1–6–12)　　图1–6–13 (Fig.1–6–13)　　图1–6–14 (Fig.1–6–14)

（6）收式（图1-6-15~图1-6-21）

当上身恢复到直立位时，双手自体侧向前外侧展出，到达肩关节高度时，两手内收至额部印堂穴使中指相接。双手合十，沿体前正中线缓缓下落。

当落至膻中穴高度时，保持两中指相接，分开两掌并使之与地面平行，缓缓下按。

当落至肚脐（神阙穴）高度时，两手自然分离，置于身体两侧。

恢复到预备式。

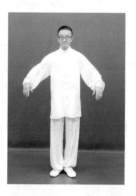 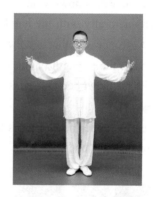

图1-6-15 (Fig.1-6-15)　　图1-6-16 (Fig.1-6-16)

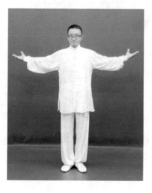 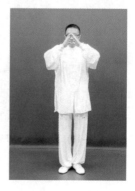

图1-6-17 (Fig.1-6-17)　　图1-6-18 (Fig.1-6-18)

(6) Closing form (Fig.1-6-15～Fig.1-6-21)

When the upper body returns to the upright position, stretch your hands forward and outward to the shoulder level so that the two hands connect at Yintang. With the hands put together, bring them down slowly along the midline in front of the body.

When the hands reach Danzhong, keep the two middle fingers connected. Hold the two palms apart and parallel to the ground. And then press them down slowly.

When reaching the navel level (Shenque), separate both hands naturally and place them alongside the body.

Return to the preparatory posture.

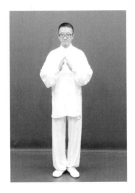 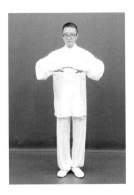

图1–6–19 (Fig.1–6–19)　　图1–6–20 (Fig.1–6–20)

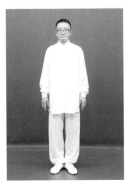

图1–6–21 (Fig.1–6–21)

2. 易犯错误

（1）展翅扩胸时，两臂不够舒展，胸部的扩张幅度不够充分。

（2）俯身下按时，双手未落到膻中穴即开始俯身，膝关节弯曲，未能挺直、并拢。

（3）攀足挺臀时，双手中指分离，掌面未能与地面平行，臀部未能向后上方挺起，致使上半身未能向双腿靠拢。

（4）垂掌竖腰时，双臂垂掌过于僵硬，竖腰未应用腰部的力量带动上身，而是直接抬头起身。

3. 操作强度

如果本节功法与全套功法一起操作，一般情况操作3次或6次。

如果单独操作本节功法，可以根据自身状况，按照3、6、9、12的次数递增运动量，最多不超过12次。

4. 功法作用

本节功法冠名"固肾腰"，就是要通过双手攀足的动作，引动足太阳膀胱经和足少阴肾经的经气运行，达到强腰固肾的作用。

在俯身下按至攀足挺臀的操作过程中，使头颈部、背部、腰部、下肢后侧的软组织受到最大限度的牵拉、伸展，能够全面有效激发足太阳膀胱的经气运行，而足太阳膀胱经"入腰中，络肾，属膀胱"，尤其攀足挺臀和垂掌竖腰对腰部的作用力更大，同时又要用腰部的力量带动整体完成整套动作，而腰部的位置处于人体的中间部位，这对改善全身气血循环非常有利。

2. Common Mistakes

(1) In the movement of spreading the arms and expanding the chest, the arms are not completely stretched out and the chest is not fully expanded.

(2) In the movement of stooping down and pressing the hands downward, it's wrong to bend over before the hands reach Danzhong. Besides, the knees are bent rather than straightened and brought together.

(3) In the movement of hands touching feet with the buttocks up, the middle fingers of both hands are separated and the palms are not parallel to the ground. The buttocks are not raised upward so that the upper body fails to move close to the two legs.

(4) In the movement of letting the palms hang down with the waist upright, the hanging arms are too stiff. Moreover, when raising the waist upright, instead of applying the strength of the waist to drive the upper body, one raises his head and rises to his feet directly.

3. Amount of Qigong Exercises

This routine, when done together with a full set of Qigong exercises, is generally done 3 or 6 times.

When doing this routine alone, you can gradually increase the amount of exercise by 3, 6, 9 or 12 times according to your own condition. Do it 12 times at most.

4. Functions and Effects

This routine, entitled "to strengthen the kidney and waist", is to strengthen the waist and the kidneys through touching the feet with the hands, which initiates the circulation of Bladder Meridian of Foot-*Taiyang* and the Kidney Meridian of Foot-*Shaoyin*.

In the process from stooping down and pressing the hands downward to hands touching the feet with the buttocks up, soft tissues in the head, neck, back, waist and hamstrings are stretched and pulled to the greatest extent so that it can effectively stimulate the circulation of the meridian qi of the Bladder Meridian of Foot-*Taiyang*. What' more, the Bladder Meridian of Foot-*Taiyang* "enters the waist, connects with the kidneys and pertains to the bladder". In particular, the movements of stooping down and pressing the hands downward and hands touching the feet with the buttocks up can exert greater strength on the waist. Moreover, the whole set of movements are completed with the assistance of the waist strength. As the waist lies in the center of the body, this routine is extremely beneficial to the qi and blood circulation of the whole body.

根据中医学理论，腰为肾之府，泌尿、生殖系统的功能都与"腰"的关系密切，因此，本节功法对此类疾病的康复有很好的作用。通过充分的向前俯身动作，能够有效地牵拉腰部、下肢后侧肌群，缓解以上部位的紧张，能够调整脊柱平衡，可以用于脊柱病的防治，同时对腹部（尤其小腹部）器官组织的作用也是直接的，能够用于妇科、男科及泌尿系疾病的调治。

第七节　攒拳怒目增气力

本节功法是在预备式的基础上，按照先左后右的顺序，左右两手交替出拳进行操作的。

1. 调身操作步骤

（1）预备式（图1-7-1、图1-7-2）

两足跟并拢，脚尖外分。双手自然垂在身体两侧，目视远方，全身放松。

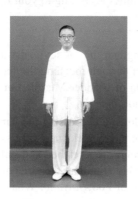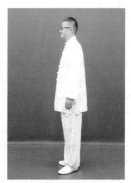

图1-7-1 (Fig.1-7-1)　　图1-7-2 (Fig.1-7-2)

（2）开步握拳（图1-7-3、图1-7-4）

右脚向外开一步半，两脚尖微微内扣，使双脚平行，站稳踏实，目视正前方。两腕关节微曲，掌心向后，指尖向下，两手沿体侧缓缓提起，至两侧髂棘高度，握成空拳（拳心向下、拳眼向内）。

According to the theory of traditional Chinese medicine, the waist houses the kidneys. The functions of the urinary and reproductive systems are closely related to the "waist". So, this routine has a very good effect on the recovery of diseases of this kind. Stooping down fully in this routine can effectively stretch the waist and hamstrings, relieve the tension in such parts and keep the spine balanced. It can be used for the prevention and treatment of spinal diseases. Besides, it bears effects directly on the abdominal organs (particularly those in the lower abdomen) and for this reason it can regulate and treat gynecological, andrological and urological diseases.

Routine 7　Thrusting the Clenched Fists Forward with Glaring Eyes to Enhance Strength

This routine is based on the preparatory posture and practiced by punching alternately with the left hand and the right hand according to the sequence of left first and then right.

1.Step–by–step Instructions

(1) Preparatory posture (Fig.1-7-1, Fig.1-7-2)

Stand with heels together and tiptoes apart. Place both hands alongside the body. Look straight ahead. Keep the whole body relaxed.

(2) Taking a step sideways and clenching the fists (Fig.1-7-3, Fig.1-7-4)

Take a big step and a half outward with the right foot. Keep the tiptoes slightly clutched inward and the two feet parallel to each other. Stand steadily and firmly on the ground. Look straight ahead. Slightly bend the two wrists with palms backward and fingertips downward. Raise both hands slowly alongside the body to the level of the iliac crest and hold them into hollow fists (with the inner sides downward and the thumb-sides inward).

两拳在髂棘平面，以两前臂纵轴为中心，向外旋转180°，旋至拳心向上、拳眼向外。

同时，两肘关节内收，肩关节下沉，呈蓄势待发之势。

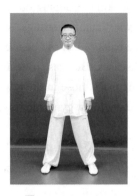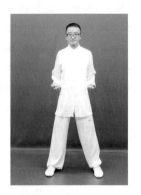

图1-7-3 (Fig.1-7-3)　　　　图1-7-4 (Fig.1-7-4)

（3）左拳后展（图1-7-5～图1-7-9）

左拳带动左臂，向后、后上画弧后展，至肩关节高度，同时，以腰为轴，上身向左、左后，缓缓磨转，目光始终锁定左拳。

然后，将左拳内收于左侧耳郭后外侧，使拳心向下、拳眼向内，左侧肘关节同时外展。

上身以腰为轴，缓缓向前、向右磨转，同时两膝关节屈曲，缓缓下蹲成马步。

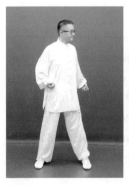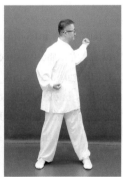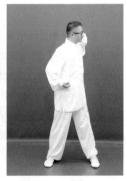

图1-7-5 (Fig.1-7-5)　　　图1-7-6 (Fig.1-7-6)　　　图1-7-7 (Fig.1-7-7)

At the level of the iliac crest, take the two forearms as the longitudinal axes and rotate the fists outward to 180° until the inner sides face upward with the thumb-sides outward.

Meanwhile, adduct the elbows and relax the shoulders. Hold a ready-to-go posture.

(3) Left fist swinging backward (Fig.1-7-5～Fig.1-7-9)

Driven by the left fist, swing the left arm backward and upward like drawing an arc till up to the shoulder level. Meanwhile, taking the waist as an axis, swing the upper body slowly to the left and the left back side with the eyes fixed on the left fist.

Then, adduct the left fist to the posterolateral side of the left auricle with the inner side downward and the thumb-side inward. Meanwhile, stretch the left elbow outward.

Taking the waist as an axis, slowly swing the upper body forward and right. Simultaneously, bend both knees and squat into a horse stance slowly.

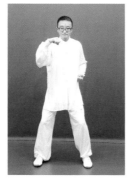
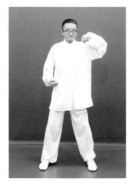

图1-7-8(Fig.1-7-8)   图1-7-9 (Fig.1-7-9)

（4）出拳怒目（图1-7-10～图1-7-13）

左拳自耳后向身体正前方出拳，至身体正前方（膻中穴高度），距离身体正中30～50cm，左腕关节悬起、左肘关节微屈。

然后，以下动作同时进行操作：紧握双拳、圆瞪双目、紧咬牙关、收紧全身肌肉，大约停顿3秒。

顺势，松力放松，左拳向外缓缓旋转、回撤至左侧髂棘处（带脉穴①），同时起身恢复到开步握拳。

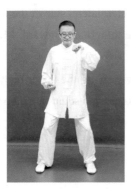 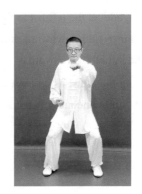

图1-7-10 (Fig.1-7-10)　　　图1-7-11 (Fig.1-7-11)

（5）右拳后展（图1-7-14～图1-7-18）

右拳带动右臂，向后、后上画弧后展，至肩关节高度，同时，以腰为轴，上身向右、右后，缓缓磨转，目光始终锁定右拳。

然后，将右拳内收于右侧耳郭后外侧，使拳心向下、拳眼向内，右侧肘关节同时外展。

① 带脉穴：属于足少阳胆经的穴位，位于第11肋骨游离端垂线与脐水平线的交点上。

(4) Punching with glaring eyes (Fig.1-7-10~Fig.1-7-13)

Thrust the left fist from behind the ear to the straight front of the body. When the fist reaches the straight front of the body (level with Danzhong), 30~50 cm apart from the body, raise the left wrist with the left elbow slightly bent.

Then, do the following simultaneously: clench the fists tightly, keep the eyes widely open, clench the teeth, tighten the muscles of the whole body and hold for about 3 seconds.

Then along with loosening up, slowly rotate the left fist outward and adduct it to the left iliac crest (Daimai[①]). At the same time, rise back to the position of "taking a step sideways and clenching fists".

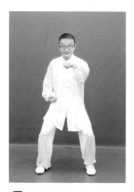 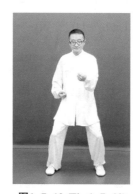

图1-7-12 (Fig.1-7-12)   图1-7-13 (Fig.1-7-13)

(5) Right fist swinging backward (Fig.1-7-14~Fig.1-7-18)

Driven by the right fist, swing the right arm backward and upward like drawing an arc till up to the shoulder level. Meanwhile, taking the waist as an axis, swing the upper body slowly to the right and the right back side with the eyes fixed on the right fist.

Then, adduct the right fist to the posterolateral side of the right auricle with the inner side downward and the thumb-side inward. Meanwhile, stretch the right elbow outward.

---

① Daimai (BG26): one of the acupoints of the Gallbladder Meridian of Foot-Shaoyang, at the intersection of the vertical line at the free end of the 11th rib and the horizontal line of the navel

上身以腰为轴，缓缓向前、向左磨转，同时两膝关节屈曲，缓缓下蹲成马步。

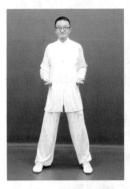 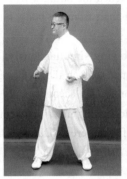 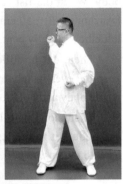

图1-7-14 (Fig.1-7-14)　　图1-7-15 (Fig.1-7-15)　　图1-7-16 (Fig.1-7-16)

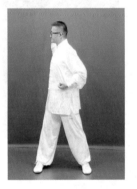 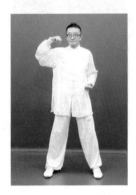

图1-7-17 (Fig.1-7-17)　　　　图1-7-18 (Fig.1-7-18)

（6）出拳怒目（图1-7-19、图1-7-20）

右拳自耳后向身体正前方出拳，至身体正前方（膻中穴高度），距离身体正中30～50cm，右腕关节悬起、右肘关节微屈。

然后，以下动作同时进行操作：紧握双拳、圆睁双目、紧咬牙关、收紧全身肌肉，大约停顿3秒。

顺势，松力放松，右拳向外缓缓旋转、回撤至右侧髂棘处（带脉穴），与此同时，上身起身恢复到开步握拳。

Taking the waist as an axis, slowly swing the upper body forward and left. Simultaneously, bend both knees and squat into a horse stance slowly.

(6) Punching with glaring eyes (Fig.1-7-19, Fig.1-7-20)

Thrust the right fist from behind the ear to the straight front of the body. When the fist reaches the straight front of the body (level with Danzhong), 30～50 cm apart from the body, raise the right wrist with the right elbow slightly bent.

Then, do the following simultaneously: clench the fists tightly, keep the eyes widely open, clench the teeth, tighten the muscles of the whole body and hold for about 3 seconds.

Then along with loosening up, slowly rotate the right fist outward and adduct it to the right iliac crest (Daimai). Simultaneously, rise back to the position of "taking a step sideways and clenching fists".

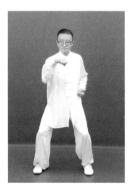 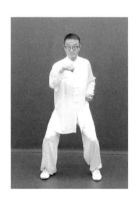

图1-7-19 (Fig.1-7-19)　　图1-7-20 (Fig.1-7-20)

（7）收式（图1-7-21～图1-7-30）

两拳放松，由拳化掌，掌心向上置于髂棘处。

两掌自下向上画圆，于头顶中指相接，掌心内合。双手合十，沿体前正中线，缓缓下落，落至肚脐高度，双手分开，置于体侧。同时重心左移，收回右脚。

恢复到预备式。

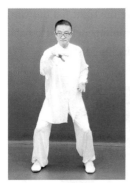
图1-7-21 (Fig.1-7-21)

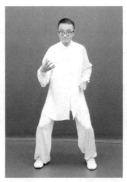
图1-7-22 (Fig.1-7-22)

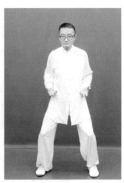
图1-7-23 (Fig.1-7-23)

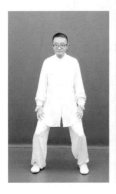
图1-7-24 (Fig.1-7-24)

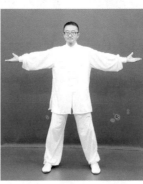
图1-7-25(Fig.1-7-25)

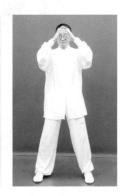
图1-7-26 (Fig.1-7-26)

(7) Closing form (Fig.1-7-21~Fig.1-7-30)

Relax the two fists and turn them into palms. Place the palms at the iliac crest with palms upward.

Circle with the two palms from bottom to top and let the middle fingers connect over the top of the head with palms inward. With the hands put together, bring them down slowly along the midline in front of the body. Keep the hands apart and place them alongside the body. Simultaneously, shift the body weight to the left and retract the right foot.

Return to the preparatory posture.

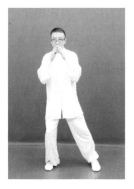
图1-7-27 (Fig.1-7-27)

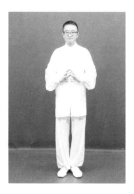
图1-7-28 (Fig.1-7-28)

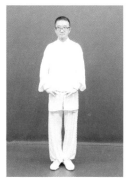
图1-7-29 (Fig.1-7-29)

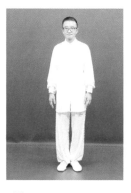
图1-7-30 (Fig.1-7-30)

2. 易犯错误

（1）拳臂后展时，上身不是以腰为轴磨转，而是髋关节出现旋转。

（2）出拳前伸时，肘关节未能充分外展，对胸胁部的牵拉不够，前伸过程中上身未能以腰为轴向右侧微微磨转，马步下蹲时出现塌腰、上身前俯等错误动作。

（3）攒拳怒目时，出现明显的耸肩、上身晃动等多余动作。

3. 操作强度

本节功法左拳怒目、右拳怒目左右交替为1次操作。

如果本节功法与全套功法一起操作，操作3次或6次。

如果单独操作本节功法，可以根据自身状况，按照3、6、9、12的次数递增运动量，最多不超过12次。

4. 功法作用

本节功法冠名"增气力"，是通过拳臂后展、出拳前伸的动作着重调动胸中之气。胸中为手厥阴心包经所起的部位、四海之一（气之海），又是宗气所聚的地方，内藏心肺两脏，胸中之气被调动起来，可以开心肺气血、通胸中气街，使气血通利，则气力可增。

2. Common Mistakes

(1) In the movement of swinging the fists and arms backward, the upper body swings with the hip joints instead of rotating with the waist as an axis.

(2) During throwing a punch, the elbows are not fully stretched outward, which causes the failure in producing a traction force enough for the chest and hypochondrium. In the process of throwing a fist forward, the upper body swings slowly to the right without taking the waist as an axis. In addition, during squatting into a horse stance, wrong movements such as the arched back and the upper body leaning forward may ensue.

(3) In the movement of clenching the fists with glaring eyes, there is an obvious shrug of the shoulders, a shake of the upper body and other unnecessary movements.

3. Amount of Qigong Exercises

In this routine, the alternative movements of the left fist with glaring eyes and the right fist with glaring eyes are counted as doing the practice for one time.

This routine, when done together with a full set of Qigong exercises, is generally done 3 or 6 times.

When doing this routine alone, you can gradually increase the amount of exercise by 3, 6, 9 or 12 times according to your own condition. Do it 12 times at most.

4. Functions and Effects

This routine, entitled "to enhance strength", lays stress on bringing qi in the chest into full play through the movements of swinging the fists and arms backward and punching out. The chest is where the Peri-cardium Meridian of Hand-*Jueyin* starts. It is one of the four seas (the sea of qi) and the place where the pectoral qi gathers and the heart and lungs are located. Regulating qi in the chest can promote the circulation of qi and blood of the two organs and connect qi pathways. As the circulation of qi and blood is promoted, qi and strength are correspondingly increased.

攒拳怒目，心"系目系"，肝"连目系"，五脏之精气皆上达于目，瞪眼怒目可以激发厥阴、少阳之气，以疏利肝胆，有效刺激交感神经兴奋，提高人体的应激性。

整套动作纵向配合马步起落，以加强气机升降；横向配合腰部磨转，以促进肾间动气，体现气的阳动之用的同时，还可加强皮肉筋骨纵横两个方向力的协调和平衡，有提高机体稳定性的临床价值。

第八节　背后七颠百病消

1. 调身操作步骤

（1）预备式（图1-8-1、图1-8-2）

两足跟并拢，脚尖外分。双手自然垂在身体两侧，目视远方，全身放松。

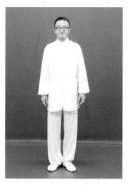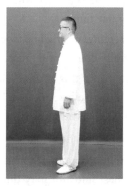

图1-8-1 (Fig.1-8-1)　　　　图1-8-2 (Fig.1-8-2)

（2）握拳提踵（图1-8-3～图1-8-5）

首先，两手自体侧向后提至腰部（大肠俞[①]平面），由掌化拳。将两拳面（四指近端指骨背侧）微微用力向前抵住腰眼[②]部。

---

① 大肠俞：属于足太阳膀胱经的穴位，位于第4腰椎棘突下，后正中线旁开1.5寸。
② 腰眼：腰背部经外奇穴，位于第4腰椎棘突下，后正中线旁开约3.5寸凹陷中。

In the movement of thrusting the clenched fists forward with glaring eyes, the essential qi of the five organs can ascend to the eyes, for the heart and the liver are associated with the eyes. Thus, glaring eyes can promote the qi of *Jueyin* (reverting yin) and *Shaoyang* (lesser yang) to soothe the liver and gallbladder, effectively stimulate the sympathetic nerves and improve the sensitivity of the body.

Cooperated with the movements of the horse stance and the waist, this Routine helps to strengthen the ascending and descending of qi and promote the dynamic qi in the kidneys. It not only embodies the functional yang of qi but also enhances the mechanical coordination and balance of flesh and bones in the vertical and horizontal directions. It is of clinical value to improve the stability of the body.

Routine 8   Raising and Lowering the Heels Seven Times to Cure Various Diseases

1. Step−by−step Instructions

(1) Preparatory posture (Fig.1-8-1, Fig.1-8-2)

Stand with heels together and tiptoes apart. Place both hands alongside the body. Look straight ahead. Keep the whole body relaxed.

(2) Clenching the fists and raising the heels (Fig.1-8-3 ~ Fig.1-8-5)

Firstly, raise both hands from the sides of the body to the waist (level with Dachangshu[①]) and change the hands from palms into fists. Exert a gentle force against Yaoyan[②] (both sides of the 4th and 5th lumbar vertebrae) with the two fists (the back sides of the proximal phalanges of the four fingers).

---

① Dachangshu (BL25): an acupoint of the Bladder Meridian of Foot-Taiyang, below the spinous process of the 4th lumbar vertebra, 1.5 cun lateral to the posterior midline
② Yaoyan (EX-B7): one of the extra acupoints on the back, below the spinous process of the 4th lumbar vertebra, in the depression approximately 3.5 cun lateral to the posterior midline

两脚足趾抓地，两腿膝关节挺直、并拢，重心微微前移。

同时，用两肘关节内收的力量微微将腰骶部向前顶出，顺势头部向后上方伸展，并引领上身向后上方伸展。然后，足跟缓缓上提，尽量离开地面，保持全身平衡、稳定，不晃动。

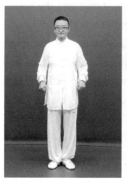 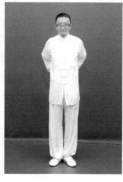 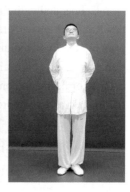

图1-8-3 (Fig.1-8-3)　　　图1-8-4 (Fig.1-8-4)　　　图1-8-5 (Fig.1-8-5)

（3）颠七振一（图1-8-6～图1-8-9）

全身协调稳定放松后，上下起落，脚跟不接触地面，均匀、缓慢地颠动7次。

在最后一次颠动足跟下落前，上身微微前移，头部恢复正直。

用全身的重力，整个身体垂直向下，快速落足，发出"咚"的振动。

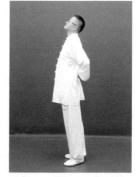

足跟落地，同时双手由拳变掌。

恢复到预备式。

图1-8-6 (Fig.1-8-6)

Clutch the ground with the toes. Hold the knees straight and the legs together. Move the body weight slightly forward.

Meanwhile, with the strength of adducting both elbows, push the lumbosacral part forward slightly. Stretch the head back and up, leading the upper body to an upward and backward extension. Then, raise the heels slowly as off the ground as possible and keep the whole body balanced and steady without shaking.

(3) Seven bounces and one vibration (Fig.1-8-6～Fig.1-8-9)

After keeping the whole body coordinated, balanced and relaxed, bounce seven times up and down at an even and slow speed with the heels not touching the ground.

Before lowering the heels in the final up-down movement, move the upper body forward a bit and get the head back to its upright position.

With the full body weight, move the whole body vertically downward and the heels to the ground rapidly with a "dong" vibration.

Bring the heels back to the ground and meanwhile change the hands from fists to palms.

Return to the preparatory posture.

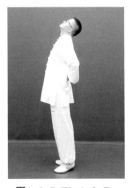 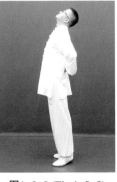 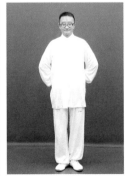

图1-8-7 (Fig.1-8-7)   图1-8-8 (Fig.1-8-8)   图1-8-9 (Fig.1-8-9)

2. 易犯错误

（1）握拳提踵中，两脚五趾未能扣紧地面、两膝关节松弛，致使重心不稳，左右、前后晃动，未能用两肘关节内收产生的力量前顶腰部，头部向后上方提伸不够，不能形成全身协调一致的态势。

（2）颠七振一中，足跟离开地面的幅度不够，颠动时左右或前后晃动，形不成全身的振荡效应。

（3）振一下落时，不够干脆、果断，形不成以一代全的纵向振动力。

3. 操作强度

如果本节功法与全套功法一起操作，一般情况操作3次或6次。

如果单独操作本节功法，可以根据自身状况，按照3、6、9、12的次数递增运动量，最多不超过12次。

4. 功法作用

本节功法冠名"百病消"，是通过全身上下颠动，产生均匀、协调的振荡波，作用于人体的气血津液，如清理水杯中的污垢一样，将体内浊气、病邪祛除。

2. Common Mistakes

(1) In the movement of clenching the fists and raising the heels, the toes fail to clutch the ground tightly and the knees are floppy, causing the body to shake from side to side or to and fro due to the instability of the center of the body weight. Moreover, the waist is not pushed forward by the strength of adducting both elbows, and the head is not fully stretched backward and upward, resulting in a poor coordination of the body.

(2) In the movement of seven bounces and one vibration, the heels are not far enough off the ground. Shaking from side to side or to and fro when bouncing the body leads to the failure in producing a vibration effect on the whole body.

(3) The one-vibration movement is done not decisively or forcefully enough to form one longitudinally vibrating strength required.

3. Amount of Qigong Exercises

This routine, when done together with a full set of Qigong exercises, is generally done 3 or 6 times.

When doing this routine alone, you can gradually increase the amount of exercise by 3, 6, 9 or 12 times according to your own condition. Do it 12 times at most.

4. Functions and Effects

This routine, entitled "to cure various diseases", is to work on qi, blood and body fluids of the body through vibrating the whole body up and down to produce even and coordinated vibrating waves. It eliminates the turbid qi and pathogenic factors just like clearing away the dirt in a water cup.

人体的经脉都是纵向分布的，足经、阴阳跷脉①、阴阳维脉②均与足部直接沟通、联系，且均上连头面，通过刺激这些经脉，可以加强气血运行，沟通上下，防患于未然；另外，由于水的比例占到人体70%以上，"水曰润下"，水的特性是向下流，通过足部颠动，振动波从下向上，加强水（尤其是血液）的回流，对改善微循环非常有效，微循环障碍又是许多慢性病的共性病理基础，长期训练对此类慢性病康复很有帮助。可见，本节功法定位百病消的用意深刻。

另外，通过振动，可以有效地放松全身各部位，并能够提高小腿后群肌力，提高人体的平衡和协调能力。

收　式

轻闭双目，搓热两手，用手心热熨眼部，如此操作3次。

---

① 阴阳跷脉：阴跷脉，起于足舟骨的后方，上行内踝的上面，沿小腿、大腿的内侧直上，经过阴部，向上沿胸部内侧，进入锁骨上窝，上行人迎（颈动脉搏动处）的上面，过颧部，至目内眦。阳跷脉，起于足跟外侧，经外踝上行腓骨后缘，沿股部外侧和胁后上肩，过颈部上夹口角，进入目内眦，再绕行头顶至枕后部。
② 阴阳维脉：阴维脉，起于小腿内侧，沿大腿内侧上行至腹部，与足太阴经相合，过胸部，与任脉会于颈部。阳维脉，起于足跟外侧，向上经过外踝，沿足少阳经上行至髋关节部，经胁肋后侧，从腋后上肩，至前额，再到项后，合于督脉。

The meridians inside the body are distributed longitudinally. Foot Meridians, Yin and Yang Heel Vessels[1] and Yin and Yang Link Vessels[2] are all connected directly with the feet and go up to the head. By stimulating these meridians, qi and blood circulation can be promoted to have a free flow up and down. Hence, various diseases can be prevented. In addition, water takes up over 70 percent in the body and is characterized by moistening and descending. In view of its features, through bouncing the feet, the down-to-up vibrating waves can strengthen the blood circulation back to the heart and effectively improve the micro-circulation. As the micro-circulation is the common pathological basis of many chronic diseases, a constant practice of this exercise is beneficial to the recovery of diseases of this kind. So, it can be clearly seen that the intention of this routine is very profound.

Moreover, the vibration can relax all parts of the body effectively, improve the strength of the posterior calf muscles and enhance the balance and coordination of the body.

Closing Form

Close the eyes gently, rub the hands together until they are very warm and then press the palms against the eyes. Repeat the process 3 times.

---

[1] Yin and Yang Heel Vessels: Yin Heel Vessel (Yin HV) is one of the eight extra meridians. It originates from the rear of the navicular bone and moves up to the inner ankle bone. It runs up along the inner side of the shank and thigh through the genital region and then continues up the medial side of the chest to emerge in the supraclavicular fossa. It proceeds up the carotid pulse through the cheekbone to the inner canthus. Yang Heel Vessel (Yang HV) is one of the eight extra meridians. It originates from the outer side of the heel and runs up the outer ankle to the posterior calf bone. Then it continues up the outer side of the thigh and the posterior hypochondriac region to reach the shoulder. It passes the neck, proceeds up the corners of the mouth to the inner canthus and then goes around the vertex of the head to the posterior or occipital region.
[2] Yin and Yang Link Vessels: Yin Link Vessel (Yin LV) is one of the eight extra meridians. It originates from the inner side of the shank and runs up the inner side of the thigh to the abdomen where it joins the Meridian of Foot-Taiyin. Then it passes the chest and reaches the neck where it joins the Conception Vessel. Yang Link Vessel (Yang LV) is one of the eight extra meridians. It originates from the outer side of the heel and runs up the Meridian of Foot-Shaoyang to the hip joint through the outer ankle. It passes the posterior side of the lateral thorax and goes up to the shoulder from the posterior armpit. Then it reaches the forehead and the back of the neck where it joins the Governor Vessel.

做完后两手十指微屈，自前额发际开始，经头顶向后，至颈后为止，轻抓头皮，反复梳理3次。

然后，上下牙轻扣9次，轻扣结束后，将舌头在口腔内壁与牙齿之间顺时针旋转9次，逆时针旋转9次，将旋转后口腔中产生的津液分3次咽下。吞咽时，注意用意念诱导津液慢慢到达小腹部，第一口缓缓地吞咽1/3下去，到达小腹部，第二口再吞咽1/3到达小腹，第三口将口中剩余的津液全部吞到小腹。

最后，搓热双手，用手掌搓腰骶部，上下搓动18次。

缓缓把双手放回体侧，睁开双眼，恢复到生活态。

Then, bend all fingers slightly. Starting at the forehead hairline, comb the scalp gently from the top of the head to the back of the neck with the bent fingers. Repeat the process 3 times.

After that, the upper teeth and the lower teeth click each other gently 9 times. Circle the tongue along the gingivae clockwise and counter-clockwise 9 times respectively between the inner wall of the mouth and teeth. Then, swallow the saliva secreted into the mouth in three gulps, 1/3 each and mentally guide it slowly to the lower abdomen.

Finally, rub the hands till they are very warm, rub the lumbosacral part with the palms and rub it up and down 18 times.

Place both hands alongside the body slowly, open the eyes and return to the daily state.

第二章　八段锦调息操作

调息操作的要领主要有以下三个方面：

第一，呼吸训练时，吸气一律使用鼻吸，呼气则可以采用鼻呼，也可以采用口、鼻同呼的方式进行操作。

第二，调息操作是建立在调身操作熟练的基础上，所以在动作训练的过程中，要学会计算各个动作的时间，以及每次吸气和呼气的时间，将动作的操作时间与吸或者呼的时间匹配起来，不断训练就会做到协调一致。

第三，如动作操作尚不熟练，在动作操作过程中，不可强迫自己过度用力吸气或呼气，可以适当地换气，或者先不要做调息操作，仍然采用我们日常的自然呼吸；而在动作操作熟练以后，逐渐再将每次吸气、呼气与相应的动作匹配起来，所以这是一个循序渐进的过程。

注意：调息的操作强度与调身相同。

第一节　两手托天理三焦

1.调息操作步骤

体侧提掌时，采用自然呼吸。

Chapter 2　Breath Adjustment Practice of Ba Duan Jin

The essentials of the breath adjustment mainly concern the following three aspects:

Firstly, during the breathing practice, breathe in only through the nose during inhalation and breathe out through the nose or through the mouth and the nose together during exhalation.

Secondly, the breath adjustment is done based on the proficient manipulation of the body adjustment. Therefore, during Qigong practice, try to learn to calculate the duration of each movement as well as the length of inhalation and exhalation each time. Only when you match the duration of each movement with that of exhalation or inhalation and practice persistently can you achieve a good coordination.

Thirdly, don't force yourself into a deep and prolonged breath during the practice if inexperienced at the practice. Instead, you can take an appropriate breath or skip the practice of adjusting the breath first and still keep breathing naturally. And when proficient in the practice, you can gradually match each inhalation or exhalation with its corresponding movement.

Tips: The exercise amount of the breath adjustment is the same as that of the body adjustment.

Routine 1　Holding Both Hands High with Palms Up to Regulate the Triple Energizer

1. Step-by-step Instructions

Breathe naturally when lifting the palms from both sides of the body.

吸气操作主要贯穿在托天提踵的动作操作过程中，使动作与吸气的时间匹配一致，具体操作是两掌托举过程缓缓吸气。注意采用鼻吸气，不可用口吸气。

当两掌上托至最高点时闭气，即不吸也不呼，初学者此时可以选择适当换气，也可以让小腹部缓慢起伏1次，以度量1个呼吸的时间。

呼气操作主要贯穿在手足同落的动作操作过程中，自两中指分离开始，至两掌落回身体两侧的整个过程，都采用呼气，主要采用鼻呼气，也可采用口鼻同呼。

注意： 如果调身操作尚不熟练，不可强迫自己进行这种深长呼吸的操作，操作过程中可以适当换气；或者先不做调息操作，仍采用自然呼吸。而在动作操作熟练后，逐渐地将每次吸气与每次托举配合起来，每次呼气与手足同落配合起来。

2. 易犯错误

过度屏气或换气，容易造成内气涩滞不通，引发胸闷气短，甚至烦躁，所以我们在练功的过程中不可过度屏气或换气。

3. 功法作用

本节功法配合平稳、柔和的呼吸运动，引动内脏协同运动，充分全面地调动三焦的气血运行，可以达到调理气血通贯上下的作用。

The inhalation mainly runs through the whole process of holding both hands high with palms up and raising the heels off the ground. The practice should match the duration of inhalation. The specific practice is to inhale slowly during lifting the palms, breathing in mainly through the nose rather than through the mouth.

When the palms are raised to the highest point, hold your breath, that is, neither inhale nor exhale. At this time beginners can choose to take an appropriate breath or measure the duration of one breath by making the slow up-down movement of the lower abdomen one time.

The exhalation mainly runs through the whole process of putting down hands and heels at the same time. From the separation of the two middle fingers to putting down the palms alongside the body, exhale mainly through the nose or through the mouth and the nose together.

Tips: Don't force yourself into a deep and prolonged breath during the practice if inexperienced at the practice. Instead, you can either take an appropriate breath or skip the practice of adjusting the breath first and still keep breathing naturally. And when proficient in the practice, you can gradually make each inhalation match each lifting movement and let each exhalation coordinate with the movement of putting down your hands and heels simultaneously.

2. Common Mistakes

Holding your breath excessively or hyperventilation may give rise to the stagnation of internal qi, resulting in a heavy sensation in the chest, shortness of breath and even vexations. For this reason, holding your breath excessively or hyperventilation should be avoided during Qigong exercises.

3. Functions and Effects

This routine, in combination with the smooth and gentle breathing movement, can stimulate the coordinated movement of the internal organs and fully promote the qi and blood circulation of the triple energizer so as to regulate the circulation of qi and blood throughout the whole body.

托举与落臂时配合呼吸，一起一落之间，呼吸深长柔细，可促进膈肌、肋间肌的协同运动，加大呼吸的幅度和深度，使更多氧气（清气）进入血液，更多的二氧化碳（浊气）排出体外，有效改善组织缺氧的症状体征，对心脑血管性疾病的预防和康复有积极作用。

第二节　左右开弓似射雕

1. 调息操作步骤

开步，转身错掌时，采用自然呼吸的方法。

吸气操作主要贯穿在下蹲开弓的动作操作过程中，使动作与吸气在时间上匹配一致。具体操作是缓缓下蹲至对抗拉弓的整个过程要缓缓吸气，此时注意采用鼻吸气，不可用口吸气。

在对抗拉弓到极致时闭气，也就是不吸也不呼，对于初学者而言，此时可以适当换气，也可以让小腹部缓慢起伏1次，以度量1个呼吸的时间。

呼气操作主要贯穿在起身合掌的动作操作过程中，自两臂松力至缓缓起身的整个过程，都采用呼气，主要采用鼻呼气，也可采用口鼻同呼。

Coordinate with respiration when lifting and dropping the arms. In between the ups and downs of breathing, keep a deep, long and soft breath. This can promote the coordinated movement of the diaphragm and intercostal muscles and increase the breathing range and depth so as to facilitate more oxygen (clear air) into the blood and more carbon dioxide (turbid air) out of the body. This can effectively improve the symptoms and signs of tissue hypoxia. It plays a positive role in the prevention and rehabilitation of cardiovascular and cerebrovascular diseases.

Routine 2   Posing as if Drawing a Bow Both Left and Right to Shoot

1. Step-by-step Instructions

Stand in a starting posture. Breathe naturally when taking a step sideways, turning around and crossing the palms.

The inhalation mainly runs through the whole process of bending the knees and drawing a bow. The practice should match the duration of inhalation. The specific practice is to inhale slowly during the process of bending the knees and drawing a bow, breathing in mainly through the nose rather than through the mouth.

When drawing the bow to an extreme, hold your breath, that is, neither inhale nor exhale. Beginners can take an appropriate breath at this time or measure the duration of one breath by making the slow up-down movement of the lower abdomen one time.

The exhalation mainly runs through the whole process of rising to your feet and putting the palms together. From loosening the arms to rising to your feet slowly, exhale mainly through the nose or through the mouth and the nose together.

注意：如果调身操作尚不熟练，不可强迫自己进行深长的调息训练，因为操作过程中会引起我们非常不舒适的感受。在操作过程中，由于我们调息的操作需要慢细匀长，所以，我们可以在操作初期做适当的换气，同时也可以先不做调息的操作，采用自然呼吸。而当动作操作熟练之后，逐渐地将每次吸气与拉弓匹配起来，呼气与我们的起身合掌匹配起来。

2. 易犯错误

动作操作尚未熟练时，强行匹配呼吸，容易造成呼吸不均匀，胸闷气喘；过度吸气或过度呼气，造成呼吸结滞，容易引起两胁肋胀痛紧张，甚至会引起情绪烦躁不安的问题。

3. 功法作用

开弓时展肩扩胸，促进呼吸肌群（主要是肋间内外肌）的力量，配合呼吸调控（主要是膈肌），可加大氧气的吸入量，以增强肺活量，加强氧气与二氧化碳的交换率，有通宣理肺，改善心肺功能之功效。

第三节　调理脾胃须单举

1. 调息操作步骤

提腕举掌时，采用自然呼吸。

吸气操作主要贯穿在整个左托右按或右托左按的动作操作过程中，使动作与吸气的时间匹配一致。具体操作是左手或右手缓缓托举到对侧手缓缓下按的整个过程采用缓缓吸气，注意采用鼻吸气，不可用口吸气。

Tips: Don't force yourself into a deep and prolonged breath during the practice if inexperienced at the practice, otherwise it may cause you to feel uncomfortable. As the practice of the breath adjustment requires a slow, even and deep breath, you can take an appropriate breath in the early stage of the practice or skip the practice of adjusting the breath first and still keep breathing naturally. And when proficient in the practice, you can gradually make each inhalation match the movement of drawing a bow and let each exhalation coordinate with the movement of rising to your feet and putting the palms together.

2. Common Mistakes

When you are inexperienced at the practice, if you force yourself to match the respiration, it may cause an uneven breath, a heavy sensation in the chest and panting. Excessive inhalation or excessive exhalation may lead to breathing stagnation, causing distending pain and tension in hypochondria and even emotional restlessness.

3. Functions and Effects

In the movement of drawing the bow, it can expand the shoulders and the chest, which can promote the strength of respiratory muscle group (mainly internal and external intercostal muscles). If cooperated with respiratory adjustment (mainly diaphragm), it can increase the oxygen intake, enhance the vital capacity, strengthen the exchange rate between oxygen and carbon dioxide, and thus have the effects of diffusing and regulating the lung qi and improving the functions of the heart and lungs.

Routine 3   Holding One Arm Aloft Alternately to Regulate the Functions of the Spleen and Stomach

1. Step-by-step Instructions

Breathe naturally when raising up the wrists and palms.

The inhalation mainly runs through the whole process of left-handed lifting with right-handed pressing or right-handed lifting with left-handed pressing. The practice should match the duration of inhalation.The specific practice is to inhale slowly during the process of lifting up with the left hand or right hand and pressing down slowly with the other hand, mainly through the nose rather than through the mouth.

在托、按至极致时闭气，即不吸也不呼，初学者在此时可以适当换气，也可以用小腹部的缓慢起伏来度量1个呼吸的时间。

呼气操作主要贯穿在左落右托或者右落左托的动作操作过程中，自托举手缓缓下落至下按手缓缓上举至肩关节高度的整个过程，都采用呼气，主要采用鼻呼气，也可采用口鼻同呼。

注意：如果调身操作尚不熟练，不可强迫自己进行深长的调息操作，操作过程也可适当进行换气。如果动作操作尚不熟练，仍采用自然呼吸。在动作操作熟练之后，逐渐使每次吸气与每次托举匹配起来。

2. 易犯错误

（1）调息操作时，由于动作不熟练，很容易出现单臂上举的操作时间大于单臂回落的时间，出现吸气操作时间大于呼气操作时间这样的问题。

（2）左托右按、右托左按时，如果过度屏气，会造成胸闷、憋气等不良反应。

3. 功法作用

单举的动作操作是外在动作，而配合呼吸以调动膈肌的升降，可以牵拉胸腔、腹腔的脏器，尤其对居于中焦的脾胃（包括大小肠等空腔脏器）能起到按摩的作用，从而促进胃肠蠕动，改善消化及代谢功能。

When lifting and pressing to an extreme, hold your breath, that is, neither inhale nor exhale. Beginners can take an appropriate breath at this time or measure the duration of one breath by making the slow up-down movement of the lower abdomen one time.

The exhalation mainly runs through the process of left arm falling with right-handed lifting or right arm falling with left-handed lifting. In the whole process from the slow fall of the lifted hand or the slow rise of the downward pressing hand to the shoulder level, breathe out mainly through the nose or through the mouth and the nose together.

Tips: Don't force yourself into a deep and prolonged breath during the practice if inexperienced at the practice. Instead, you can take an appropriate breath or skip the practice of adjusting the breath first and still keep breathing naturally. And when proficient in the practice, you can gradually make each inhalation match the movement of each lifting and pressing.

2. Common Mistakes

(1) During the adjustment of the breath, due to the lack of proficiency, raising up the arm may cost more time than putting down the arm so that the inhalation lasts longer than the exhalation.

(2) In the movement of left-hand lifting with right-hand pressing or right-hand lifting with left-hand pressing, holding the breath excessively is likely to induce such adverse reactions as a heavy sensation in the chest, suffocation and so on.

3. Functions and Effects

Holding one arm aloft is an external movement. If assisted by the adjustment of the breath, it can motivate the ups and downs of the diaphragm and pull the internal organs in the chest and abdomen and have a massage effect on the spleen and stomach in particular (including the hollow organs such as the large and small intestines) in the middle energizer, which can promote the gastrointestinal peristalsis and improve digestive and metabolic functions.

第四节　五劳七伤往后瞧

1. 调息操作步骤

开步，左撑右贴或右撑左贴时，采用自然呼吸。

吸气操作贯穿在整个转腰侧屈的操作过程中，使动作与吸气的时间匹配一致，即操作开步站稳后，进行转腰侧屈动作的同时要采用缓缓吸气，此时采用鼻吸的方式，不可用口吸。

转腰侧屈到最大幅度时闭气，即不吸也不呼，初学者此时可以适当换气，也可以让小腹部缓慢起伏1次，以度量1个呼吸的操作时间。

呼气操作主要贯穿在起身回掌的动作操作过程中，自起身回转至正立位开始，到两掌落回身体两侧的整个过程，都采用呼气，主要采用鼻呼气，也可采用口鼻同呼。

注意：如果调身操作尚不熟练，不可强迫自己进行深长的呼吸锻炼，操作过程中可以适当换气；或者先不做调息操作，仍在自然呼吸的基础上进行动作操作。而当动作操作熟练后，逐渐使每次吸气和每次撑、贴及转腰侧屈的动作配合起来。

2. 易犯错误

本节功法在调息操作时，吸气与呼气的速度太快，呼吸急促，容易造成胸闷、憋气等不良反应。

Routine 4   Looking Backward to Relieve Five Consumptions and Seven Impairments

1.Step-by-step Instructions

Take a step sideways with one foot, shoulder-width apart. Breathe naturally during pushing the left arm forward with the right arm against the back or pushing the right arm forward with the left arm against the back.

The inhalation mainly runs through the process of turning the waist and bending sideways. The practice should match the duration of inhalation. The specific practice is to inhale slowly during the whole practice of turning the waist and bending sideways, mainly through the nose rather than through the mouth at this moment.

When turning the waist and bend sideways to its maximum limitation, hold your breath, that is, neither inhale nor exhale. Beginners can take an appropriate breath at this time or measure the duration of one breath by making the slow up-down movement of the lower abdomen one time.

The exhalation mainly runs through the process of turning the body back to the midline and adducting the palms. From turning the body back to the midline to putting down the palms alongside the body, exhale mainly through the nose or through the mouth and the nose together.

Tips: Don't force yourself into a deep and prolonged breath during the practice if inexperienced at the practice. Instead, you can take an appropriate breath or skip the practice of adjusting the breath first and still keep breathing naturally. And when proficient in the practice, you can gradually make each inhalation and exhalation match the movement of each pushing, pressing as well as turning the waist and bending sideways.

2. Common Mistakes

During the practice of the breath adjustment, the rapid inhalation and exhalation are likely to induce such adverse reactions as a heavy sensation in the chest, suffocation and so on.

3. 功法作用

本节功法调息着重在转腰侧屈操作时，配合吸气，一方面增加腹腔压力可以激发小腹部的丹田①之气，而呼吸停闭又进一步使这个压力作用进一步持续；另一方面整个动作是以腰骶椎为支点旋转的，吸气使动作产生的外部旋转力转换成内在螺旋力，对内部任脉、督脉和冲脉的气血起到回旋提升的效应，结合后续的缓缓呼气，以起到张弛有度的疗伤作用。

第五节　摇头摆尾去心火

1. 调息操作步骤

开步俯身，采用自然呼吸。

吸气操作贯穿在整个左撑右按或右撑左按至摇头摆尾的操作过程中，使动作与吸气的时间匹配一致。具体操作是右撑左按或左撑右按，头摇向后上方，尾骨摆向对侧后方的整个过程缓缓吸气，此时注意采用鼻吸气，不可用口吸气。

---

① 丹田：指炼丹产丹的部位，为人体之本，真气汇聚之地，练功意守之处。分为上丹田（眉心位置）、中丹田（两乳头连线的中点）、下丹田（在脐下3寸，小腹正中线）。

3. Functions and Effects

The emphasis of the breath adjustment in this routine is laid on the cooperation between turning the waist and bending sideways and inhalation. On the one hand, the increased abdominal pressure can stimulate the qi of Dantian[①] (elixir field) in the lower abdomen while holding the breath enables this pressure to continue further. On the other hand, the whole movement rotates with the lumbar vertebrae as a supporting point. The inhalation turns the external revolving force generated by this routine into an internal spiral force, which has a positive effect on the improvement of the qi and blood circulation of the Conception Vessel, Governor Vessel and Chong Vessel. Coordinated with the subsequent slow exhalation, it can achieve a proper healing effect.

Routine 5   Swinging the Head and Lowering the Body to Eliminate Stress-induced Heart Fire

1. Step-by-step Instructions

Breathe naturally when taking a step sideways and stooping down.

The inhalation mainly runs through the whole process from "left arm pushing and right-handed pressing or right arm pushing and left-handed pressing" to "swinging the head and lowering the body". The practice should match the duration of inhalation. The specific practice is to inhale slowly during the movements of "right arm pushing and left-handed pressing or left arm pushing and right-handed pressing" and "swinging the head backward and upward while lowering the body and turning it to the other side". Remember to inhale mainly through the nose rather than through the mouth at this moment.

[①] Dantian: Dantian (elixir field, 丹田 dān tián) refers to the place for producing Dan (the elixir) in alchemy, where the root of the human body lies, genuine qi is stored and the mind is focused in Qigong exercises. Dantian is divided into the upper Dantian (between the eyebrows), the middle Dantian (at the midpoint of the line connecting the nipples) and the lower Dantian (3 cun below the navel in the midline of the lower abdomen).

摇头摆尾至最大限度时闭气，即不吸也不呼，初学者此时可以适当换气，也可以让小腹部缓慢起伏1次，以度量1个呼吸的时间。

呼气操作主要贯穿在松力回旋至对侧转身的动作操作过程中，自头部松力开始，至俯身磨转至正前方，接着进行对侧转身的整个过程，都采用呼气，主要采用鼻呼气，也可采用口鼻同呼。

注意：如果调身操作尚不熟练，不可强迫自己进行深长的呼吸操作，操作过程中可以适当换气；或者先不做调息操作，在自然呼吸的状态下进行动作训练。而在动作操作熟练后，逐渐使每次呼吸与每个动作匹配起来。

2. 易犯错误

调息操作时，吸气与呼气的速度太快或呼吸急促，可引起胸闷、憋气的症状。

3. 功法作用

在躯体伸展、旋转的动作训练过程中，配合深长柔细的呼吸运动，对调节体内气血的升降出入和内脏的协调功能有很好的作用。

第六节　两手攀足固肾腰

1. 调息操作步骤

预备式，采用自然呼吸。

When swinging the head and lowering the body to your maximum limitation, hold your breath, that is, neither inhale nor exhale. Beginners can take an appropriate breath at this time or measure the duration of one breath by making the slow up-down movement of the lower abdomen one time.

The exhalation mainly runs through the whole process of loosening and adducting to turning the body to the other side. The whole practice starts from loosening the head to turning the body to the straight front, then to the other side. Remember to breathe mainly through the nose or through the mouth and the nose together.

Tips: Don't force yourself into a deep and prolonged breath during the practice if inexperienced at the practice. Instead, you can take an appropriate breath or skip the practice of adjusting the breath first and still keep breathing naturally. And when proficient in the practice, you can gradually make each inhalation and exhalation match each corresponding movement.

2. Common Mistakes

During the practice of the breath adjustment, the rapid inhalation and exhalation are likely to induce a heavy sensation in the chest and suffocation.

3. Functions and Effects

The practice of the body extension and rotation in this routine, combined with a deep, long and soft breathing movement, has a good effect on the regulation of the ascending, descending, exiting and entering of qi and blood in the body and the coordination between the internal organs as well.

Routine 6   Moving the Hands Down and Touching the Feet to Strengthen the Kidney and Waist

1. Step-by-step Instructions

Breathe naturally in the preparatory posture.

吸气操作贯穿在展翅扩胸的动作操作过程中，使动作与呼吸的时间匹配一致。具体操作是当预备式站稳后，两臂外展，开始吸气，此时注意采用鼻吸气，不要采用口吸气，一直到两手中指相合于印堂穴的高度时。

呼气操作贯穿在俯身下按的动作操作过程中，自印堂穴高度至双手下按至足面的过程，整个过程都采用呼气，主要是鼻呼气，也可以采用口鼻同呼。

攀足挺臀，当感觉到足跟部受到牵拉，此时开始闭气，即不吸也不呼，初学者此时可以适当换气，也可以让小腹部缓慢起伏1次，以度量1个呼吸停闭的时间。

此外，在垂掌竖腰时吸气，竖腰完成后呼气，恢复预备式接下一次操作。

注意：如果调身操作尚不熟练，不可强迫自己进行深长的呼吸操作，操作过程中可以适当换气；或者在自然呼吸的基础上完成调身操作。

2. 易犯错误

吸气与呼气的速度太快、太急，不能与操作的动作协调匹配，容易造成呼吸和动作的匹配不当，引起胸闷、憋气、气短、胁肋胀痛等症状。

3. 功法作用

本节功法对每次吸气和呼气训练的时长要求都很高，展翅扩胸配合吸气，能够有效牵拉肺组织、提高肺活量；俯身下按、攀足挺臀配合呼气乃至呼吸停闭，能够加大肺中浊气的排出量，使气血向身体远端流通。两者协同，能够提高肺的通气功能，加强腰部气血循环，改善脑供血和远端肢体微循环。

The inhalation mainly runs through the process of spreading the arms and expanding the chest. The practice should match the duration of inhalation. After standing firm in the preparatory posture, the specific practice is to spread the arms outward and begin to inhale until the two middle fingers meet at Yintang. Remember to breathe in mainly through the nose rather than through the mouth at this moment.

The exhalation mainly runs through the process of stooping down and pressing the hands downward. Exhalation starts from Yintang to pressing both hands till touching the back of the feet. Breathe out mainly through the nose or through the mouth and the nose together.

In the process of hands touching the feet with the buttocks up, hold your breath when you feel a pulling force from the heels, that is, neither inhale nor exhale. Beginners can take an appropriate breath at this time or measure the duration of one breath by making the slow up-down movement of the lower abdomen one time.

Besides, inhale when letting the palms hang down with the waist upright and then exhale after completing it. Return to the preparatory posture and continue from the next practice.

Tips: Don't force yourself into a deep and prolonged breath during the practice if inexperienced at the practice. Instead, you can take an appropriate breath during the practice or complete the practice of adjusting the body based on breathing naturally.

2. Common Mistakes

The rapid inhalation and exhalation may result in the failure to coordinate with the corresponding movements, causing a heavy sensation in the chest, suffocation, shortness of breath and distending pain in hypochondria.

3. Functions and Effects

This routine has a demanding requirement for the duration of each inhalation and exhalation. The cooperation with inhalation in the movement of spreading the arms and expanding the chest can effectively pull the tissues of the lungs and improve the lung capacity; the coordination with exhalation or even holding your breath in the movements of stooping down while pressing the hands downward and hands touching the feet with the buttocks up is of great help to discharge the turbid qi out of the lungs and to push qi and blood to the distal end of the body. Both can improve the respiratory function of the lungs, the qi and blood circulation of the waist, the cerebral blood supply and the distal limb microcirculation.

第七节　攒拳怒目增气力

1. 调息操作步骤

开步握拳时，采用自然呼吸。

吸气操作贯穿在左拳后展或右拳后展的操作过程中，使动作与吸气的时间匹配一致。具体操作为开步站稳后握拳，左拳后展或右拳后展整个过程采用缓缓吸气，此时注意采用鼻吸气，不可用口吸气。

呼气操作贯穿在出拳过程中，具体操作是出拳至身体正前方的过程中采用缓缓呼气，主要采用鼻呼气，也可以采用口鼻同呼。

出拳至身体正中线时闭气，同时紧握双拳、瞪圆两目、咬紧牙关、收紧全身肌肉，大约停顿3秒。

收拳恢复到预备式，采用自然呼吸。

2. 易犯错误

吸气与呼气的速度太快、太急，不能与动作协调配合，容易造成呼吸急促、胸闷、憋气等问题。

3. 功法作用

本节功法吸气、呼气分别随展臂、出拳动作及身体的起落完成，一方面促进机体内在的脏腑气血与远端肢体经络之气沟通；另一方面闭气伴随短暂紧张状态，能够兴奋交感神经系统，提高内脏运动的协调功能。

Routine 7   Thrusting the Clenched Fists Forward with Glaring Eyes to Enhance Strength

1. Step-by-step Instructions

Breathe naturally when taking a step sideways and clenching the fists.

The inhalation mainly runs through the process of swinging the left or right fist backward. The practice should match the duration of inhalation. The specific practice is to clench the fists after standing firm in the starting posture and inhale slowly when swinging the left or right fist backward. Breathe in mainly through the nose rather than through the mouth.

The exhalation mainly runs through the process of thrusting the fists forward. The specific practice is to exhale when thrusting the fists to the front of the body, breathing out mainly through the nose or through the mouth and the nose together.

When thrusting the fists to the front of the body, hold your breath for about 3 seconds, clenching the fists, glaring the eyes and tightening the muscles simultaneously.

Retract the fists, return to the preparatory posture and breathe naturally.

2. Common Mistakes

The rapid inhalation and exhalation may result in the failure to coordinate with the corresponding movements, causing shortness of breath, a heavy sensation in the chest and suffocation.

3. Functions and Effects

In this routine, each inhalation or exhalation is done respectively along with stretching the arm, punching and the rise and fall of the body. On the one hand, it can promote the communication between the qi and blood of internal organs and the meridian qi of the distal limbs; on the other hand, holding the breath accompanied by momentary tension can stimulate the sympathetic nervous system and improve the coordination of the movement among the internal organs.

第八节　背后七颠百病消

1. 调息操作步骤

预备式时，采用自然呼吸。

吸气操作主要贯穿在握拳提踵的动作操作过程中，使动作与吸气的时间匹配一致。具体操作是两手提至腰部，抵住腰眼，足趾抓地，重心前移，足跟抬起的整个过程采用缓缓吸气，注意采用鼻吸气，不可用口吸气。

当脚尖站稳后闭气，即不吸也不呼，同时上下起落，足跟不着地，颠动7次。

呼气操作主要贯穿在足跟落地的动作操作过程中，最后一次颠动，用全身重力快速落足，接触地面，发出"咚"的声音后，双手顺势松开变掌的同时呼气，主要采用鼻呼气，也可采用口鼻同呼。

注意：如果调身操作尚不熟练，不可强迫自己进行如此的呼吸操作方法，操作过程中可以适当换气；或者先不做调息操作，仍采用自然呼吸。在动作操作熟练后，逐渐使每次呼吸与动作匹配起来，尤其是吸气与握拳提踵匹配起来。

2. 易犯错误

吸气与呼气的速度太快、太急，配合动作不协调，虚颠7次时不能做到闭气，造成气力松懈。

3. 功法作用

本节功法将呼吸训练应用到身体上下振荡的运动中，能够从纵向疏通身体上下的气血，可以有效清理体内浊气，达到调和阴阳、延缓衰老的功效。

Routine 8   Raising and Lowering the Heels Seven Times to Cure Various Diseases

1. Step-by-step Instructions

Breathe naturally in a preparatory posture.

The inhalation mainly runs through the process of clenching the fists and raising the heels off the ground. The practice should match the duration of inhalation. The specific practice is to raise the hands up to the waist and press them against Yaoyan. Inhale slowly in the whole process of clutching the ground with the toes, moving the body weight forward and raising the heels off the ground. Remember to breathe in through the nose rather than through the mouth.

After standing firm on the tiptoes, hold your breath, that is, neither inhale nor exhale. At the same time, bounce seven times up and down with the heels off the ground.

The exhalation mainly runs through the process of lowering the heels to the ground. In the final up-down movement, let the heels rapidly down to the floor with the full body weight. Following a "dong" sound, loosen the hands from fists into palms. At the same time, exhale mainly through the nose or through the mouth and the nose together.

Tips: Don't force yourself into a deep and prolonged breath during the practice if inexperienced at the practice. Instead, you can take an appropriate breath or skip the practice of adjusting the breath first and still keep breathing naturally. And when proficient in the practice, you can gradually make each inhalation and exhalation match the corresponding movement, especially let each inhalation coordinate with the movement of clenching the fists and raising the heels.

2. Common Mistakes

The rapid inhalation and exhalation may result in the failure to coordinate with the corresponding movements. In addition, in the up–down movement for seven times with the heels off the ground, the failure in holding the breath induces the slackness of qi and strength.

3. Functions and Effects

In this routine, the breathing practice is applied to the up-down vibrating movement of the body. It is conducive to a free flow of the internal and external qi and blood of the body longitudinally, effectively cleans up the turbid qi in the body and achieves the yin-yang harmony and anti-aging process.

第三章　八段锦调心操作

调心操作的要领有以下四个方面：

第一，根据各节功法设定的具体内容进行调心的操作，八段锦主要选择了存想①和意守②两个意念性的操作内容，要合理、有效地调动自身的感知觉与相应的动作、呼吸进行匹配。

第二，调心操作是在调身和调息操作熟练的基础上来进行的，所以要在动作和呼吸操作熟练之后，再加意念操作，才能进行有效的调心训练。

第三，意守和存想的强度不宜太大，不可猛想猛练，意识要轻柔和缓，怡然自得。

第四，坚持训练，循序渐进，才能将调心操作的内容匹配到相应的动作和呼吸当中，做到无痕对接。

注意：调心的操作强度与调身相同。

---

① 存想：亦称存思，是想象特定的景物至清晰可见、身历其境状态的心理操作活动，内观某一物体的形貌、活动状态等，以期达到集中思想，去除杂念，进入气功境界。
② 意守：将意念集中和保持在身体某一部位或某一事物上的方法和过程，通过意守可排除杂念，实现"一念代万念"，逐步达到气功入静状态。

Chapter 3　Mind Adjustment Practice of Ba Duan Jin

The essentials of the mind adjustment include the following four aspects:

Firstly, the adjustment of the mind is done in accordance with the specific contents set by each routine. Ba Duan Jin (An Eight-Routine Invaluable Qigong Exercise) mainly covers the practice of Yi Nian (guided mind or ideas/thoughts in the mind) including Cun Xiang[①](inward contemplation) and Yi Shou[②] (mind concentration). It is necessary to mobilize your sensation and perception rationally and effectively to match the corresponding movement and respiration.

Secondly, the mind adjustment is done based on the proficient adjustments of the body and breath. Therefore, the guided mind practice should not be added until you are skilled at the movement and respiration. Only in this way can you proceed to the training of the mind adjustment in an effective way.

Thirdly, the practice of mind concentration and inward contemplation should never be excessive nor violent. Be gentle and at ease with the mind.

Fourthly, a step-by-step and persistent practice is required. Only in this way can you make the adjustment of the mind match the corresponding movement and respiration to achieve a perfect coordination.

Tips: The exercise amount of the mind adjustment is the same as that of the body adjustment.

---

① Cun Xiang (存 想 cún xiǎng): inward contemplation or inward thinking, a mental training process of keeping the mind on imagined specific scenes till to be clearly visible and visualizing the shape and active state of an object or a scene in order to get rid of distracting thoughts and become tranquil

② Yi Shou (意守 yì shǒu): mind concentration, a method and process of concentrating and keeping the mind on a certain object or a specific body part, which can help to remove distracting thoughts, replace the ten thousand thoughts with one single thought and gradually become meditative.

第一节　两手托天理三焦

1. 调心操作步骤

托天提踵时，存想双手如托起一块巨石，缓缓自体侧向体前向上托起。当上托至头顶时，存想与巨石的压力进行对抗，以伸展我们整个躯体。

呼吸停顿时，存想巨石已被送入天际而消解，感觉自己从足到头顶逐渐贯通而舒展。

手足同落时，两臂如大鹏展翅，缓缓下落，如释重负，全身放松，引气下行，归于足跟。

2. 易犯错误

存想时，一是用意太过、火候太强；二是意念与动作、呼吸的匹配不协调，顾此失彼，容易造成精神紧张，不能有效放松。

3. 功法作用

用存想取重物的一念，托举负重，展臂释重，能够有效消除内心压力和杂念，举重若轻，对改善心源性疲劳有促进作用。

Routine 1   Holding Both Hands High with Palms Up to Regulate the Triple Energizer

1. Step-by-step Instructions

When holding the hands high and raising the heels, visualize holding up a huge rock with the hands and lifting it slowly from the lateral sides to the front of the body. When lifting it over the head, visualize fighting against the pressure of the huge rock to stretch the whole body.

When holding your breath, visualize yourself sending the huge rock into the sky to vanish there, feeling a gradual stretch from the heels to the top of the head.

When putting down the hands and heels simultaneously, stretch both arms like a roc spreading its wings and then let them down slowly as if you were greatly relieved. Relax the whole body and guide qi down to the heels.

2. Common Mistakes

During the inward contemplation, the first is the mental overconcentration and excessive practice. The second is that the guided mind is unable to be coordinated with its movement and respiration. It is liable to cause mental stress and failure in an effective relaxation.

3. Functions and Effects

Taking a heavy object with the guided mind, bearing weights when lifting and releasing from weights when stretching the arms can effectively eliminate mental pressure and distracting thoughts, which can promote the improvement of cardiogenic fatigue.

第二节　左右开弓似射雕

1. 调心操作步骤

转身错掌时，存想后手空拳如捏紧弓弦，前手化爪如握弓身。

下蹲开弓时，存想后手空拳如捏弓弦而后拉，同时前手如爪握弓身向前上方用力推弓，意想①弦紧弓沉，力从腰背而起，马步扎稳，上身向后倾斜，眼神从握弓手处看向前上方如瞄准前上方翱翔的大雕。

呼吸停顿时，蓄势待发，静待猎物。

起身合掌时，存想箭射雕落，弦回弓松。全身放松，如释重负，引气归原，归于小腹。

2. 易犯错误

意识昏沉造成动作散漫，不能将整个动作操作梳理成取弓与箭、弓箭搭扣、对抗拉弓、瞄准射雕这样的整体心理操作过程。

3. 功法作用

存想开弓射雕的心理操控过程，有助于促进心身融合，以导气令和、通融机体左右气血平衡。

---

① 意想：用意想象的感知觉操作，也就是存想。

Routine 2 Posing as if Drawing a Bow Both Left and Right to Shoot

1. Step-by-step Instructions

When turning around and crossing the palms, visualize clenching the bowstring with one hand in a hollow fist position and holding the bow with the other hand in a claw-like position.

When squatting and posing as if drawing a bow, visualize drawing the bowstring backward with one hand in a hollow fist position and at the same time forcefully pushing the bow forward and upward with the other hand as if holding the bow. Picture to yourself [①] the bow is fully bent and very heavy. Exert the strength from the lower back. Keep the horse stance steady. Tilt the upper body backward and look forward and upward along the hand holding the bow, as if aiming at an eagle flying up above in the sky.

Hold your breath and visualize yourself waiting for a prey and an opportunity to shoot.

When rising to your feet and putting the hands together, visualize yourself releasing the arrow to shoot an eagle down and then bringing the bowstring back to position with the bow loosened. Relax the whole body as if you were greatly relieved and guide qi down to the lower abdomen.

2. Common Mistakes

The drowsy mind may give rise to a loose and disorganized movement. As a result, the entire movement cannot be sorted into the mental controlling process of taking a bow and arrow, placing the arrow on the string, drawing the bow with the opposite strength and aiming to shoot an eagle.

3. Functions and Effects

The mental controlling process of drawing a bow to shoot an eagle is conducive to the integration of the mind and body, the harmony achieved by guiding qi and the balance of qi and blood at both sides of the body as well.

---

① Yi Xiang (意 想 yì xiǎng): imagined sensation and consciousness, also known as inward contemplation or inward thinking

第三节 调理脾胃须单举

1. 调心操作步骤

手掌举按时，存想托举之手如托起巨石，缓缓自体侧向前上托起，当托至头顶时，存想与巨石的压力对抗。存想下按之手如压水中浮木，时时与浮力对抗。

呼吸停顿时，存想巨石被送入天际而消解，浮木被压入水中，沉入水底。

左落右托或右落左托时，全身放松，如释重负，存想落手时像大鹏展翅缓缓落下。

2. 易犯错误

意识散漫、不集中，不能有效调控姿势和动作的协调性，左右两侧的托举与回落不一致，不协调，对清气与浊气升降的存想不够细腻，不能诱导出真实的内在感受。

3. 功法作用

应用意念的主动调控，存想托举时清气升腾，回落时浊气下降，双臂对抗时清气在体内回旋以濡养脏腑器官，更能促进脾胃气化、内气运转，为除百病奠定基础。

Routine 3　Holding One Arm Aloft Alternately to Regulate the Functions of the Spleen and Stomach

1. Step-by-step Instructions

When lifting one hand and pressing down the other one, visualize lifting the hand as if lifting a huge rock slowly from the side to the front of the body. When holding it over the top of the head, visualize fighting against the pressure of the huge rock. When pressing down the other hand, visualize pressing a driftwood into water and fighting against the buoyancy constantly.

Hold your breath and visualize yourself sending the huge rock into the sky to vanish there and pressing the driftwood into water, down to the bottom of water.

In the movement of left arm falling with right-handed lifting or right arm falling with left-handed lifting, relax the whole body as if you were greatly relieved and visualize putting down the hand in the way a roc spreads its wings to fly downward slowly.

2. Common Mistakes

The distraction of mind or the lack of concentration may lead to the failure in an effective adjustment of the postures and a good coordination of the movements as well as the inconsistence of lifting up and putting down the hands at both sides. The inward contemplation of the spleen and stomach's function of ascending the lucid and descending the turbid is not in great detail. Therefore, it can't induce the true inner feelings.

3. Functions and Effects

With the active control of the guided mind, visualize the ascending of clear qi when lifting the hands, the descending of turbid qi when putting down the arms and the circulation of clear qi to nourish *zang-fu* organs when exerting opposite strength with both arms. It can promote the qi transformation of the spleen and stomach and the qi circulation in the body, which can lay a foundation for the elimination of various diseases.

第四节　五劳七伤往后瞧

1. 调心操作步骤

左右撑贴时，意识集中到腰部被手贴放的位置，细细地感受，细细地品味。

转腰侧屈时，意识深入到腰内部，随着侧屈下降至足心。

呼吸停顿时，细细地感受足心受到挤压的感觉。

起身回掌时，感觉气血沿原路回到腰部。

2. 易犯错误

调心操作时，意守强度太大，注意力过度集中而不放松。

3. 功法作用

本节功法采用意守操作，将意念从脑海中转移到肢体末端的相应部位、穴位上，有催动气血通灌四肢百骸以疗外伤的效用；最后引导气血回到腰部，以疗内伤。

Routine 4   Looking Backward to Relieve Five Consumptions and Seven Impairments

1. Step-by-step Instructions

During pushing the left arm forward with the right arm against the back or pushing the right arm forward with the left arm against the back, concentrate the mind on the waist where the hands are placed and feel it with your heart.

During turning the waist and bending sideways, keep the mind deep into the waist and then down to the soles along with the lateral bending of the upper body.

Hold your breath and feel carefully how the soles react when pressed firmly.

While turning the body back to the midline and adducting the palms, guide the qi and blood back to the waist along the original route.

2. Common Mistakes

In adjusting the mind, the mind is too concentrated to be relaxed, which induces a mental overconcentration.

3. Functions and Effects

This routine is to transfer the guided mind to the corresponding locations and acupoints at the end of the extremities by means of the mind concentration, which has an effect of promoting the circulation of qi and blood all through the extremities and bones to treat external injuries. Finally, it guides the qi and blood back to the waist to treat internal injuries.

第五节　摇头摆尾去心火

1. 调心操作步骤

摇头摆尾时，意守整个脊柱，细细感受从颈椎、胸椎、腰椎到尾椎的旋转过程。

呼吸停顿时，意守尾骨尖端（即俗话所说的尾巴骨）。

松力回旋时，全身放松，意守下丹田。

2. 易犯错误

调心操作时，意守强度太大，或过于集中，没有意识到摇头摆尾是通过头部带动、引动脊柱的整体旋转，最后力点应该集中在尾骨区域。

3. 功法作用

调心操作将意念守护到脊柱，引导气血沿脊柱，从上向下至尾骨，能够疏通督脉经气，醒神开窍，益气养神。

Routine 5   Swinging the Head and Lowering the Body to Eliminate Stress-induced Heart Fire

1. Step-by-step Instructions

While swinging the head and lowering the body, keep the mind on the whole spine, and feel with your heart the rotation from the cervical vertebrae to the thoracic vertebrae, then to the lumbar vertebrae and finally to the caudal vertebrae.

While holding your breath, keep the mind on the apex of the caudal bone (namely tailbone in colloquial language).

During the loosening and adducting movements, relax the whole body and keep the mind on the lower Dantian.

2. Common Mistakes

In adjusting the mind, the mind is too concentrated or there is a mental overconcentration, failing to realize that it is the head that actually drives the whole spine to swing and rotate in the movement and finally the point of strength should be focused on the caudal vertebrae.

3. Functions and Effects

In the practice of adjusting the mind, defending the spine by keeping the mind on it and then guiding the qi and blood to the tailbone from top to bottom along the spine can unblock the meridian qi of the Governor Vessel, refresh the mind, replenish qi and nourish the spirit.

第六节　两手攀足固肾腰

1. 调心操作步骤

展翅扩胸提掌时，存想自小腹丹田处有一股内气或暖流向上提到胸部，随展臂流向两掌。

俯身下按时，双掌再引气下行。

攀足挺臀时，存想气至足心。

呼吸停顿时，细细感受足心的变化。

垂掌竖腰时，双掌引气回到小腹。

2. 易犯错误

意识引导气血运行的操作过快，不能与缓慢的动作协调一致，容易造成意气分离。

3. 功法作用

意念调动丹田内气通行身体上下，再从足底涌泉穴[①]引气入腹，有引火归原，濡养肾气之效。

---

① 涌泉穴：属于足少阴肾经的穴位，位于足心最凹陷处，约足底第2、3跖趾缝纹头端与足跟连线的前1/3与后2/3交点上。

Routine 6　Moving the Hands Down and Touching the Feet to Strengthen the Kidney and Waist

1. Step-by-step Instructions

In the movements of stretching the arms, expanding the chest and lifting the palms, visualize a flow of warm qi from Dantian in the lower abdomen up to the chest and then to the palms along with stretching the arms.

In the movement of stooping down and pressing the hands downward, guide qi down with both palms.

In the movement of hands touching the feet with the buttocks up, visualize a flow of qi to the soles.

Hold your breath and feel carefully how the soles react.

In the movement of palms hanging down with the waist upright, guide qi with both palms back to the lower abdomen.

2. Common Mistakes

The practice to guide the circulation of qi and blood with the mind is done too fast to coordinate with the slow movements, resulting in the separation of the mind from qi.

3. Functions and Effects

This routine has an effect of guiding fire back to its origin and nourishing kidney qi by means of using the guided mind to motivate the circulation of qi within Dantian throughout the body and then lead qi into the abdomen from Yongquan[①] in the soles.

---

① Yongquan (KI1): an acupoint of the Kidney Meridian of Foot-Shaoyin, in the depression of the sole, at the junction of the anterior third and posterior two-thirds of the line connecting the base of the 2nd and 3rd toes and the heel

第七节　攒拳怒目增气力

1. 调心操作步骤

拳臂后展时，眼随手走，意在拳心。

出拳怒目时，意灌于力，气力相合，发劲迅猛，全身紧张。

旋拳回撤时，骤然放松，力解气不散，眼随手走，气与意合。

收拳起身时，气自胸中沿任脉，缓缓向下回归小腹下丹田。

2. 易犯错误

意识引导气血运行的操作过快或间断，不能与缓慢的动作协调一致，造成意气的分离。

3. 功法作用

意气相随，气与力合，张弛有度，有益气行气、疏肝理气的功效。

Routine 7   Thrusting the Clenched Fists Forward with Glaring Eyes to Enhance Strength

1. Step-by-step Instructions

In the movement of swinging the fists and arms backward, the eyes move with the hands, keeping the mind on the inner sides of the fists.

In the movement of punching with glaring eyes, infuse the mind into force, combine qi with strength, exert a rapid and hard force and keep the whole body tightened.

In the movement of rotating and retracting the fists, get relaxed all of a sudden. Force is released but qi still gathers together. The eyes move with the hands and qi goes along with the mind.

In the movement of retracting the fists and rising to your feet, bring the qi slowly from the chest back to Dantian in the lower abdomen along the Conception Vessel.

2. Common Mistakes

The practice to guide the circulation of qi and blood with the mind is done too fast or discontinuous to coordinate with the slow movements, resulting in the separation of qi from the mind.

3. Functions and Effects

In this routine, the mind goes along with qi while qi combines with strength, which can replenish qi, promote qi circulation, soothe the liver and regulate qi.

第八节　背后七颠百病消

1. 调心操作步骤

握拳提踵时，双拳顶腰，存想头上有一绳子向上牵拉，全身被提起，仅脚尖着地。

颠七振一时，虚颠7次，细细感受全身如水纹上下震动的感觉。

振一下落，存想体内振荡出来的浊气随呼气被全部排出体外。

2. 易犯错误

意识松懈，不能将存想内容有效发挥，尤其是颠动时产生意识涣散。

3. 功法作用

意念与颠七振一操作相配合，诱导全身经络气血随"颠动"畅达，以振奋全身阳气，祛除百病。

Routine 8   Raising and Lowering the Heels Seven Times to Cure Various Diseases

1. Step-by-step Instructions

When clenching the fists and raising the heels off the ground, place the fists against the waist and visualize an invisible string over the head and pulling it straight up so that the whole body is lifted up, only with the tiptoes on the ground.

In the movement of seven bounces and one vibration, raise and lower the heels seven times off the ground and feel the up and down vibration like water waves in the whole body with your heart.

When doing the one-vibration movement, visualize expelling the turbid qi through the vibration out of the body along with each exhalation.

2. Common Mistakes

The mind is too relaxed to bring what are in the inward contemplation into full play effectively, especially during the bouncing movement, leading to the distraction of mind as a result.

3. Functions and Effects

The mutual coordination between the guided mind and the movement of "seven bounces and one vibration" can induce a free flow of the meridian qi and blood of the whole body along with "bounces and vibrations" so as to stimulate yang qi and eliminate various diseases.

后 记

　　本书将以调身为主的八段锦功法的学习和训练过程，按照调身、调息、调心的顺序进行安排，目的在其外部动作、姿势训练熟练的基础上，再引导大家将这些动作与相应的呼吸操作、心理训练匹配起来，逐渐强化练功的内在体验，进而达到三调合一①的气功境界目标，使我们的身与心融合成一个整体，以契合《素问·上古天真论》所倡导的"形与神俱，而尽终其天年，度百岁乃去"的健康养生理念。

　　本套八段锦功法是在中医学传统理论的指导下，结合西医学的原理，进行整理的医学气功动功功法，适应人群比较广泛，各节功法组合在一起对人体身心的训练既有整体效应，又有各自相对的独立性和针对性。虽然本书匹配了相应的图片以帮助大家练习，但仍然可能会有不易掌握的细节。遇此之时，请大家登录中国大学MOOC、学习强国App等网站平台，搜索北京中医药大学《中医气功学导论》课程，注册登录后，会有更多直观学习本套八段锦的机会（配有中英文字幕），也可以通过该慕课的课堂讨论区进行咨询和交流。

---

① 三调合一：三调是指调身、调息、调心；三调合一是通过坚持、重复的训练，将三者融合为一个有机整体的操作过程，也指身心融合的气功境界状态。

Epilogue

This book, with a focus on the body adjustment, presents readers in great detail about how to learn and practice Ba Duan Jin (An Eight-Routine Invaluable Qigong Exercise). In the sequence of the body adjustment, the breath adjustment and the mind adjustment, it guides readers step by step to make each movement coordinate with its corresponding practice in the breath adjustment and the mind adjustment based on the skilled practice of external movements and postures. It can gradually strengthen the internal experience and then reach the Qigong state of the "Three Adjustments integrated into one"[①]. It is conducive to the integration of our body and mind into a whole, which happens to conform to the health and life-nurturing concepts advocated in *Plain Questions· Ancient Ideas on How to Preserve Natural Healthy Energy* (Sù Wèn ·Shàng Gǔ Tiān Zhēn Lùn, 素问 · 上古天真论), " (Therefore, they could maintain) a desirable harmony between the *Shen* (mind or spirit) and the body, enjoying good health and a long life."

Under the guidance of traditional Chinese medical theory and the principles of Western medicine, this set of Ba Duan Jin has been sorted into a kind of dynamic exercise of medical Qigong, which is adaptable for a wide range of people. The combination of all the routines has either an overall effect or its relative independence and pertinence. Although the relevant illustrations in the book can help you with your practice, there are still some details that you may find difficult to grasp. For more information, please log in to the website platfoms of China Universities MOOC (Massive Open Online Courses) (中国大学 MOOC), Learning Power App(学习强国App) and so on, then search the course entitled *Introduction to Chinese Medical Qigong* (中医气功学导论) at Beijing University of Chinese Medicine. After registration and log-in, there will be more learning opportunities for you to watch the video of this set of Ba Duan Jin (with Chinese-English captions). Moreover, consultation and communication are available through MOOC classroom discussion board.

---

① Three Adjustments integrated into one (三调合一 sān tiáo hé yī): The three adjustments refer to the body adjustment, the breath adjustment and the mind adjustment; The "Three Adjustments integrated into one" is a process of integrating the three into an organic whole through the persistent and repetitive practice, which also indicates the Qigong state of the integration of the mind and the body.

参考文献
References

［1］白彦荣，李金龙.八段锦历史源流的研究［J］.当代体育科技，2014，4(36)：208–209，211.

［2］李家晗.八段锦的历史源流与养生原理研究［D］.北京：中国中医科学院，2019.

［3］郭郁，魏玉龙，魏泽仁，等.八段锦"调心"效应对大学生"意境作业"操作的影响［J］.中医学报，2020，35(5)：1081–1087.

［4］郭郁，王卫卫，魏泽仁，等.基于α频带脑电功率谱分析八段锦诱发的不同性别大学生"调心"效应差异［J］.中华中医药杂志，2018，33(6)：2377–2382.

［5］周正坤，张彪，胡庆川，等.医学气功八段锦的功法述略［A］.世界医学气功学会（World Academic Society of Medical Qigong）.世界医学气功学会第五届理事会第二次会议暨第八届学术交流会议论文集［C］.北京：世界医学气功学会，2014：168–172.

［6］刘天君，章文春.中医气功学［M］.北京：中国中医药出版社，2016.

［7］魏玉龙.中医气功实训教程［M］.北京：中国中医药出版社，2014.

［8］李照国，刘希茹.汉英气功学大辞典［M］.上海：上海科学技术出版社，2020.

［9］庄子（战国），James Legge（英国）.英汉双语国学经典 理雅各英译本《庄子》［M］.郑州：中州古籍出版社，2016.

［10］The Chinese Health Qigong Association. Chinese Health Qigong: Ba Duan Jin ［M］.Beijing: Foreign Language Press, 2008.

［11］James MacRitchie. Health Essentials: Cultivating Personal Energy–Chi Kung ［M］. UK: Element Books Limited Lonmead, Shaftesbury, Dorset, 1993.

［12］谢竹藩，谢方. 新编汉英中医药分类词典 ［M］.北京：外文出版社，2019.

［13］Judith Farquhar, Qicheng Zhang. Nurturing Life in Contemporary Beijing–Ten Thousand Things ［M］. USA: Zone Books, 2012.

［14］孙慧，曹玉麟. 基础中医英语 ［M］.青岛：中国海洋大学出版社，2010.

［15］Paul U. Unschuld. The Classic of Difficult Issues ［M］. USA: University of California Press. 2016.

［16］李照国，刘希茹. 大中华文库汉英对照黄帝内经·素问 ［M］. 西安：世界图书出版公司. 2005.

［17］李照国，刘希茹. 大中华文库汉英对照黄帝内经·灵枢 ［M］. 西安：世界图书出版公司. 2008.

［18］Tianjun Liu, Kevin W Chen. Chinese Medical Qigong ［M］. London and Philadelphia: Singing Dragon, 2010.

［19］上海市气功研究所. 中医气功常用术语词典 ［M］. 上海：上海科学技术出版社，2015.

［20］张仲景，李照国，刘希茹. 汉英对照金匮要略 ［M］.上海：上海三联书店，2016.

［21］Nigel Wiseman, Feng Ye. A Practical Dictionary of Chinses Medicine ［M］.Second Edition, Fourth Printing. Massachusetts: Paradigm Publications, 2002.